The Hospice Companion

The Hospice Companion

Best Practices for Interdisciplinary Care of Advanced Illness

Third Edition

Perry G. Fine, MD

Professor of Anesthesiology
Pain Research Center
School of Medicine
University of Utah
Salt Lake City, Utah

Associate Editor

Matthew Kestenbaum, MD

Capital Caring
Washington, DC

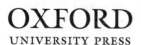

OXFORD
UNIVERSITY PRESS

OXFORD
UNIVERSITY PRESS

Oxford University Press is a department of the University of Oxford. It furthers
the University's objective of excellence in research, scholarship, and education
by publishing worldwide. Oxford is a registered trade mark of Oxford University
Press in the UK and certain other countries.

Published in the United States of America by Oxford University Press
198 Madison Avenue, New York, NY 10016, United States of America.

© Oxford University Press 2016

First Edition Published in 2008
Second Edition Published in 2012
Third Edition Published in 2016

Library of Congress Cataloging-in-Publication Data
Names: Fine, P. G. (Perry G.), editor. | Kestenbaum, Matthew, editor.
Title: The hospice companion : Best practices for interdisciplinary care of advanced illness/
[edited by] Perry G. Fine ; associate editor, Matthew Kestenbaum.
Description: Third edition. | Oxford ; New York : Oxford University Press, [2016] | Includes
bibliographical references and index.
Identifiers: LCCN 2016006944 | ISBN 9780190456900 (alk. paper)
Subjects: | MESH: Hospice Care—methods | Palliative Care—methods | Patient Care Team |
Terminally Ill—psychology | Handbooks
Classification: LCC R726.8 | NLM WB 39 | DDC 362.17/56—dc23 LC record available at
http://lccn.loc.gov/2016006944

9 8 7 6 5 4 3 2

Printed by Webcom, Inc., Canada

Acknowledgments

This third edition of *The Hospice Companion* reflects labors of love by an experientially rich and dedicated cohort of professionals from Capital Caring, a premier advanced illness coordinated health-care system providing hospice and palliative care services throughout the metropolitan Washington, DC area. Their work is possible only due to the visionary and courageous leadership of this organization's Chief Executive Officer, Malene Davis: visionary, because of her foresight to see the necessity of high-quality comprehensive services that extend far beyond the last days of life for people living with chronic progressive illnesses; courageous, because of her willingness to take significant risks, break away from conventional and limited models of care, insist on measuring what matters most, *never* deny needed care to *anyone* for *any* reason, support education for the next generation of hospice and palliative medicine specialists, partner with traditional health-care systems in novel and innovative ways, develop a research enterprise to advance the field, and prove that this can and must be done within a sustainable economic model. And last, but far from least, we are immeasurably grateful for the trust of the many families who open their doors to us each and every day, and allow us the privilege of being of service, which propels us ever forward in our individual and collective evolution as a civil society—where each of us is stronger for the dignity we help each other achieve throughout the entirety of our lives.

The editors, authors, and contributors would like to extend special thanks and appreciation to the Washington Hospital Center Library staff for their expertise and invaluable assistance in helping with literature searches.

Foreword

We all have deeply personal stories about the serious illness and eventual loss of people whom we loved and cared deeply about. Everyone has a story. I have one about my father.

These stories endure. And they can weigh heavily on us, often for the wrong reasons. We think about—sometimes are haunted by—the thoughts of seemingly needless and avoidable suffering we have witnessed at life's end. Sometimes we may feel that we inadvertently helped to cause or sustain the suffering, or could have somehow prevented it. If only . . .

I have my father's powerful story, and I also have others, because many people have entrusted me with their tales of what it is like for loved ones to die in America. They do this—from U.S. Senators to nurses to old college friends to casual acquaintances—because I am involved with C-TAC, the Coalition to Transform Advanced Care.

Most of these stories are about what could have been done better for people who were seriously ill. Through these narratives and through many professional experiences, I have concluded that we <u>must</u> improve our culture and systems of care. Our current approach to treating advanced illness and the end of life is simply unsustainable. Moreover, it is wrong. Our approach often violates the dignity and the values of the dying. And beyond that, the physical and emotional toll on caregivers and surviving family members is painful and lasting.

Clearly, it is time to transform advanced illness care.

Research into the essential wants and needs of people facing life-limiting illness is remarkably consistent, regardless of how different each of us and our individual circumstances may be. These wants and needs are often surprisingly simple and attainable, if only we understand what they are and make them a priority.

What are they? Three basic things:

- To be at home, and eventually to die with family, friends and other loved ones present if at all possible;

- To have pain and other symptoms managed effectively, which allows for attention to more meaningful matters, including spiritual needs; and

- To ensure that families are not financially and emotionally devastated by the experience of a loved one's illness and death.

We can attain all this. But to meet these goals of care, fundamental changes are necessary. Our current approach is based not on compassion or logic so much as inertia and habit. It is deeply rooted in acute models of care and payment structures, rather than preferences and values.

This makes change exceedingly difficult, but it can be done. And together, we can make it happen. The first step in *fixing* the problem, as has often been said, is to *understand* the problem.

It's important to note that we are making progress. We have reached the threshold of understanding. Most people—health professionals, policy makers and the public—are coming to realize that we clearly have a problem. And it is a very large one, considering our rapidly aging population, soaring health care costs and patient and family dissatisfaction with the way things are.

Now what? Can we muster the courage, the political will, the gumption and collective intelligence to say "enough is enough?" I believe we can, and I believe we will.

One of my favorite quotes, from the mathematician Piet Hein, comes to mind at this point: "Problems worthy of attack, prove their worth by attacking back." This is just such a problem, big and complex, and one that doesn't lend itself to sitting on our hands and waiting for change to happen. We need to fight the problem on four fronts:

• To engage the public. This means informing patients, caregivers and families to help them understand what they are confronting; to think about and document their preferences and values, as well as their available options and the potential consequences of their choices; and to enable people to communicate their wishes to doctors and nurses and others who are involved in their treatment.

• To better prepare and support our clinicians, and to provide them with the skills and tools they need to do right by their patients.

• To take what is working now and create best practice models of care to promote throughout all of our health systems.

• To advocate effectively for policy changes at state and national levels— legislative and regulatory—to align payment and incentives, research, education and support toward improving care.

The Hospice Companion is an important book. It is encouraging and insightful, and it fuels my optimism that we are making progress. Dr. Perry Fine has given healthcare professionals a powerful tool to address and mitigate the almost overwhelming burdens experienced by their very sick and dying patients and their families.

This book is a best practices and evidence-based guide for clinicians and other health professionals on how to address the many biomedical, social, psychological and spiritual aspects of advanced illness. It is a practical approach that paves the way to greatly improve the outcomes that matter most at a very vulnerable time for everyone involved.

Perry Fine has provided a critical step to transform advanced illness care; one that every clinician can and must take to meet his or her professional and ethical obligations and to make a difference in people's lives.

The rest is up to all of us . . . "to fight back" and to win.

Bill Novelli
Bill Novelli is a professor at the McDonough School of Business at Georgetown University, where he leads the Global Social Enterprise Initiative. He is also co-chair of the Coalition to Transform Advanced Care (C-TAC) and was previously CEO of AARP.

Preface

With the "Boomers" passing the torch to the "Millennials," the next and third generation of health-care professionals to enter the workforce since the inception of hospice care in America, it would have been both apt and timely to call this *The Hospice Companion, Third Generation.* Much as we look up to, honor, and respect those who trust us to provide their care as they come to the end of their lives, so, too, do we strive to pass along our hard-won experience and wisdom from one generation to the next. In a nutshell, this is the aspirational goal of *The Hospice Companion.*

And it was really only so recently in this history of American health care that, with the simple stroke of a pen, one of the most remarkable developments in modern health care occurred: the enactment of the Medicare Hospice Benefit—just in time to establish a better model of end-of-life care for the "Greatest Generation." This public policy development was an acknowledgment that hospital-based care for the dying was discordant with essential human needs at this unique time in the life cycle and that there was a reasonable economic alternative. But for just as long, I have called this the "best-kept secret in American health care" because still, after more than three decades, far too few people—including doctors as well as patients and their loved ones—understand the extraordinary value of this all-inclusive service: value that can be measured both in terms of well-defined and highly desirable clinical outcomes and dollars. After the fact, those who do obtain hospice care often ask, "Why didn't we learn about this earlier?" It's a good question, and one whose answer lies in ever-evolving cultural change.

Even though more and more people with life-limiting diseases are connecting with hospice care, there remain hundreds of thousands who die in the United States with all-too-brief or complete absence of the benefit of hospice's focus on comfort, family support, dignity, peace, joy, and grace. The initial conception of *The Hospice Companion* was spurred by comparing and contrasting the scientific and structured approach that is the hallmark of modern medicine and the heartfelt and often spiritually driven paradigm of hospice care.

Based on my observations, the treatment of dying patients in hospital settings seemed to lack heart. The drive to diagnose and treat (with often futile attempts at cure) seemed to put organ systems so markedly into the foreground that the person (and his or her family and social sphere) were all but hidden—rarely to be discovered or appreciated in the course of disease management. Conversely, both the exigent (sometimes referred to as "legacy" hospices) community-based hospice programs and the rapidly growing movement toward corporate chain-based hospice programs seemed to lack the rigor of measured self-inspection and outcomes reporting. Both are necessary; neither is sufficient on its own to advance the field of advanced illness care (including end-of-life care) nor to attend to the toll that severe, progressive, and life-limiting illness takes on the body, mind, and spirit. Both are needed, and since most of us want to complete our lives in familiar surroundings (wherever we call "home"), and because the acute care model of the contemporary hospital is both anathema to the optimal end-of-life experience as well as inordinately expensive, I submit that there is no reason why "hospice heart" and "hospice mind" cannot be fostered and intertwined. Yet, empirically based scientific advancements and salutary minimization of unwarranted variability in clinical care delivery—especially around pain and symptom management—have been slow to develop within hospice. Bridging this divide was the motivation for publishing the first edition of *The Hospice Companion* after its inception as a clinical manual to provide uniform standards for a hospice provider system 20 years ago.

As with the second edition of this book, I have been graced with the help of extraordinary colleagues at Capital Caring, led by Dr. Matt Kestenbaum, all of whom sacrificed personal time and applied diligence and effort to perform literature reviews and provide their collective decades of "bedside" experience in order to update each and every chapter. The ongoing editorial challenge continues to be in keeping this book up to date and relevant to the many clinical circumstances that will likely confront hospice clinicians, without adding length and heft. It is not meant to be a comprehensive textbook. It is designed to be an easy-to-navigate, engaging, highly useful clinical decision support tool, with portability, usability, and applicability as its chief attributes.

We trust that you will find credibility and authority in the recommendations put forth in this book and that it will serve you well in your professional role, enhancing your knowledge, skills, and confidence. But in the end, it is our deep and abiding hope that reference to the third generation of *The Hospice Companion* will markedly and measurably improve the lives of those who cross paths with you. The seeming paradox brought to light in each revision of this book bears repetition: "It will be through disciplined clinical conformity and uniformity of practice that individual epiphany may have the chance to be realized as we meet our earthly ends."

Thank you for your service, your commitment, your fealty—to your profession and to your fellow man.

Perry G. Fine, MD

Contents

Contributors

Note: All contributors were full-time staff at Capital Caring, Washington DC at the time of their literature and content reviews in preparation of this edition.

Gayle Byker, MD

Carol Chang, MD

Farrah Daly, MD

John W. Dunkle, MD

Ray Jay Garcia, MD

Danielle F. Grandrimo, MD

Diane W. Hazzard, MSW

Matthew Irwin, MD

Micki Kantrowitz, MD

Jordan Keen, MD

Natalie Kontakos, MD

Jennifer Lee, DO

Dona Leskuski, DO

Laila A. Mahmood, MD

J. Cameron Muir, MD

Ann Navarro-Leahy, MD

Brenan Nierman, LCSW

Clint Pettit, MD

Michael Reynolds, MD

Mary C. O'Rourke, MD

Imran Shariff, MD

Muhammad Siddiqui, MD

Anne Silao-Solomon, MD

Jason Sobel, MD

Malgorzata Sullivan, MD

Section 1

General Processes

Palliative Care at the End of Life: Blending Structure and Function

From Information to Care

The overarching purpose of this manual, reflecting the essential goals of hospice, is to help maximize the quality of living and dying of patients during the last phase of life. With due regard for the complexities of peoples' lives, especially during severe illness, it is premised that identification and understanding of discrete situations (intertwined and enmeshed as they may be) will promote the elaboration of a care plan that will have the greatest likelihood of meeting these worthy ends.

A sequential system of reasoning and problem solving is required, and this has been devised using a standardized format throughout each subsection related to symptom management (Section 3). To accommodate the interdisciplinary nature of hospice care and promote use of this manual by all members of the interdisciplinary team (IDT), headings have purposefully been chosen that reflect a common language for all disciplines. In full appreciation of the complex and irreducible nature of human dying, an organized structure is nonetheless useful to define the mechanics and fundamentals of hospice care and the overall goal of making high-quality interdisciplinary care during the last phase of life the rule, rather than the exception.

The overall schema is summarized below. This is followed by an elaboration of terms and concepts used throughout *The Hospice Companion*.

It is recognized that variables such as advanced stage of disease at the time of hospice admission, often with very short survival times, may severely curtail the range of services that might otherwise be useful to patients and families if they had the benefit of an earlier referral with a resultant longer length of stay. In many cases, the processes of care in this book might appear to be idealized because so many patients are referred to hospice just before they die. Therefore, the full range of evaluation, assessment, and interventions proposed may need to be changed in order to hone in on the highest priorities of the patient and family to meet their most pressing needs before death. At the time of admission, attention to the likely longevity of the patient (i.e., prognosis) needs to be well considered so that the issues and goals elaborated in this guide might be realistically and specifically tailored to the needs and attainable goals of each and every patient.

Regardless of a patient's life expectancy, the most productive and "patient-centric" place to start, maintain, and deepen a trust-based relationship is with the question, "What matters most?" perhaps followed by, "What is disturbing your peace?" In those rare instances when a patient is in crisis (e.g., pain or dyspnea out of control; seizure; hemorrhaging; severe agitation/psychosis) and the cause of distress is completely obvious, urgently instituted treatment to bring the condition under control takes precedence. Otherwise, the only way to know "what matters most" and "what is disturbing your peace" is to calmly, compassionately, and openly inquire.

The flowchart "Basic Steps: Taking Care of People Who Are Dying, and Doing It Well" (Fig. 1.1) depicted in this section defines the essential steps that need to be followed, or at least considered, in the process of caring for patients at the end of life. It also serves as a teaching tool and reminder of the fundamental goals of patient-centered care within a larger system of health care. Last, it should help unravel the complex nature of the care system, clearly defining steps along the way that lead to successful patient outcomes and professional gratification.

The role of hospice is to deliver the most effective end-of-life care in the most efficient manner possible to all dying patients.

Principles of Effective Care

- The patient defines what help is needed and wanted. However, counseling about what is possible and realizable is critically important because many patients and families will be unaware of the scope of hospice services.
- As a hospice professional, know what you can contribute to accomplish these goals.
- Know whom to call upon when you reach the limits of your capabilities.
- Think and act positively. "Can't" or "won't" is not helpful.
- Actively listen: this is a powerful tool for understanding others, validating people's needs to be understood, and planning and providing care.
- Define *benefits* and *burdens* for each proposed therapeutic intervention (note: advising, counseling, and taking a "watch-and-wait" approach are all forms of an "intervention" and in this vein should be viewed in equal regard as medical treatments), remembering that there are distinct points of view: patient, family, other caregivers, professional staff, and other "stakeholders" (e.g., payers). Ask and answer: What is each party hoping for? What are the underlying motivations?
- *Benefits* and *burdens* are context-driven, requiring a full understanding of each patient's clinical and social circumstances. Determine in advance how benefits and burdens will be assessed, how often, and by whom. If *burdens* can be anticipated (e.g., constipation from an opioid analgesic), how can they be minimized in order to amplify benefits?
- Set priorities by determining which issues are most pressing.

Principles of Efficient Care

- Time is the most precious commodity we have. It must be allocated wisely and well.
- More goods (durable medical equipment, supplies, drugs), in and of themselves, do not equal better service or care. Determine what and how much of these items are necessary to accomplish the patient's goals, and continually reevaluate if they are doing what is intended.

Evaluation/Assessment
- Tools - history (all sources, including past medical records) (80% of overall time/effort)
  - physical exam (15+% of overall time/effort)
  - labs, imaging, other tests (<5% of overall time/effort)

↓

Understanding
- Patient
- Context of Patient and Family
- Family

↓

Articulation and Documentation of Realistic/Attainable Goals Taking into Account Major Stakeholders' Needs, Requirements and Expectations
- Patient
- Family
- System
  - referring physician
  - payer
  - patient's health-care network or system

↓

Development of Care Plan: First the Patient, Then the Family
- Physical Symptoms
- Practical Needs
- Psychosocial and Spiritual Needs

↓

Everything We Do Is an Intervention

Medical	**Non-Medical**	
- Additional Evaluation	- Practical Care	➡ **Defines Staffing Requirements**
- Diagnosis/Prognosis	- Interdisciplinary Team Care	(i.e., Human Resources, FTEs)
- Procedures/Prescriptions for symptom management		

↓

Thoughtful Consideration of Benefits and Burdens Anticipated and/or Resulting from Our Interventions: Discuss These at the Interdisciplinary Team Meeting

↓

Outcomes
- Measurement and Documentation of Outcomes of Interventions
- Analysis of Results

↓

Refine, Revisit, Reassess, Improve
- Is the plan working? If not, why not? How can this be remedied?

Reiterate the Process, Revising the Plan of Care Around the Goal of Optimizing the Following Quality of Life Domains and End-Outcome Measures

- QOL Domains
  - Physical symptoms and functions
  - Intrapersonal dimensions (e.g., mood, sense of hope)
  - Interpersonal status (e.g., relationships)
  - Transcendent issues (e.g., sense of meaning)
- Outcomes
  - Safe and comfortable dying
  - Self-determined life closure
  - Effective coping with imminent loss/bereavement

Figure 1.1 Basic steps of how to care for people who are dying: a logical progression of hospice case management.

• Clinical managers/leaders should cross-train and schedule human resources wisely. Determine how members of the IDT can meet patient/family goals, both to utilize their unique skills and to distribute work in an equitable and optimal fashion.

Terminology and Organizational Elements Used in Sections 2 and 3 of This Manual

Sections 2 and 3 of this manual will be structured in a similar manner as a means of reinforcing interdisciplinary, comprehensive care. Depending upon relevance, most, but not all, sections will include every dimension of assessment and process of care.

Situation

Every patient/family comes to hospice with unique attributes, clinical circumstances, and social contexts. The process of elucidating those situations that affect the well-being of each patient/family is critical to the provision of good care.

Causes

Most troublesome situations encountered by hospice patients/families can be traced to a single dominant cause or multiple contributory causes. These causes usually stem from one or more of the following domains:

• Practical (i.e., environmental, financial)
• Biomedical (i.e., disease-induced or treatment-related etiology)
• Psychosocial (i.e., related to interpersonal or intrapersonal issues)
• Spiritual (although not always easily defined in words, spiritual concerns often revolve around issues of one's sense of purpose, existence, or meaningfulness, in life and after death)

For the purposes of this guide, causes will be identified for those medically induced symptoms for which a differential diagnosis is important in the consideration of medically specific treatments.

These listings of causes are not meant to be all-inclusive but rather to provide the leading or first-line and secondary causes for most symptoms.

Findings

Findings are those elements (usually *symptoms* [patient report] and *signs* [information obtained by observation or examination]) that define or accompany any given situation and may help to identify the cause(s) of that situation. Findings are also categorized as Practical, Biomedical/Physical, Psychosocial, or Spiritual. These findings serve to identify, direct, and focus processes of care.

Assessment

The initial and ongoing determinations of Psychosocial, Biomedical/Physical, and Spiritual findings involve information gathering from one or more of the following three basic domains:

• History

Information obtainable from all sources (medical records, interviews with patient, family members, other caregivers) is far and away the most time-consuming and important part of evaluation.

- Physical Examination

This component of assessment involves observation of patient, family, and environment and hands-on examination of the patient. Albeit essential for accurate diagnosis, physical examination also links the patient and caregiver through human touch, which has therapeutic value in and of itself. Needless to say, only skilled and appropriately licensed clinicians should be involved in physical examination of the patient.

- Diagnostic Studies (blood work, imaging, other)

These types of corroborative studies are often unnecessary in order to provide high-quality palliative care at the end of life; however, there are circumstances where clinical impressions derived from history and physical examination are insufficient to formulate a well-conceived care plan. Under these circumstances, the potential benefits need to be weighed against the actual or likely burdens.

Processes of Care
The interventions listed within this section define those actions that might be taken by the IDT in order to meet patient/family needs and goals, identified through sufficient assessment.

Goals and Outcomes
Establishing goals at the outset aligns the patient/family/hospice team and promotes the monitoring of the most relevant outcomes. By explicitly stating goals, the IDT can continually assess the value of the work being done, and determine if the plan of care is appropriate. Anticipating eventualities and putting contingency plans into place are critically important to delivering high-quality end-of-life care. Ideally, outcomes will match the goals that are identified. In other words, the closer outcomes are to goals, the more successful hospice care has been.

Documentation in the Medical Record
Guidance is provided in the crucial areas of Initial Assessment, Interdisciplinary Team Notes, and IDT Care Plan in order to promote concise and pertinent recordkeeping. Thoughtful consideration of what needs to be documented serves the dual purposes of meeting regulatory compliance standards and helping the IDT to continually rethink and revisit issues that arise or are likely to arise in the context of any given patient/family system.

The Practical, Biomedical, Psychological, and Spiritual Dimensions of the Human Experience
The many inseparable dimensions of the human experience cannot be so readily categorized or unintegrated, especially under the circumstances of facing the end of one's life. As important as it may be to acknowledge this, it is equally important to identify and meet the various needs and attainable goals of dying patients and their families, with the hope that each individual can find meaning and value in his or her life as that life comes to a close. From this pragmatic starting point, four axes, or dimensions, have been used in *The Hospice Companion* to sort out and understand the nature of FINDINGS, ASSESSMENT, and PROCESSES OF CARE. **It is critically important for the IDT to understand that**

these dimensions do not delineate lines of inquiry or intervention by specific disciplines but rather those facets of the patient's or family's experience for which discrete aspects of the Care Plan can be formulated and carried out and outcomes can be measured.

Practical

These are the everyday, fundamentally important things that surround our lives, most of which we take for granted while we are healthy and able to care for ourselves.

Biomedical

This aspect of end-of-life care addresses the impact of disease on the human body and those tools that modify, reverse, slow, or palliate the progression and consequences of these biological processes. A depth of clinical knowledge, judgment, and experience is needed to understand and appropriately apply modern medical interventions in ways that will best serve the various needs and goals of patients at this stage in their life.

Psychosocial

Psychological, emotional, and social issues constitute the intrapersonal and interpersonal nature of human existence. These issues are highly complex even under the least stressful circumstances and become the focus of most need once physical symptoms are brought under control. Attention to these issues in ways that speak to the needs of dying patients and their families is implicit to quality hospice care.

Spiritual

Ultimately, one's sense of connection, meaning, purpose, or value within the greater scheme of things is most likely to rise to the surface when confronting mortality. Attention to this uniquely human concern, at the pace and within the framework of the patient/family ethos, presents a truly marvelous opportunity for everyone involved and distinguishes hospice care from other alternatives within the health-care system.

Balancing Benefits and Burdens of All Interventions

Because assessment and treatment approaches offer a mixture of possible benefits and burdens to the patient, which vary depending upon each patient's circumstances, considerable thought is needed to determine the best means to optimize benefits, while minimizing burdens. The following stepwise outline should facilitate this process (see Fig. 1.2).

First

Prior to all medical procedures, all psychosocial or diagnostic tests, prescriptions, and spiritual care interventions:

- Find out "what matters most" to the patient and her/his family and "what is disturbing their peace."
- Understand pathophysiology and prognosis of ongoing disease.
- Understand family structure, support, beliefs, culture, and community ties.
- Consider the range of options for palliation of symptoms tailored to the medical/social context of the patient.
- Consider comorbidities and impact of treatment choices.

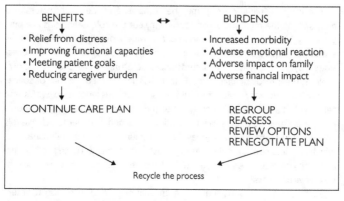

Figure 1.2 Assessing benefits and burdens.

Second

- Discuss plans and options with patient, family, and referring physician in the context of patient's needs and goals.
- Anticipate and discuss benefits and burdens.
- Initiate preventive strategies to minimize likely burdens (e.g., drug-related side effects).

Third

- Monitor and assess impact of intervention.
- Weigh benefits versus burdens over time and modify plans accordingly.
- As time passes, circumstances and priorities change and evolve, so it bears repeating on a regular basis to inquire, "What matters most now?" and "What is disturbing your peace now?"

The Interdisciplinary Team (IDT)

The Functional Hospice IDT

While there are many elements that contribute to an exceptional hospice, the IDT is at its core. In fact, the interdisciplinary rather than multidisciplinary nature of hospice is what distinguishes it from conventional health-care delivery structures. The more typical multidisciplinary group of health-care professionals functions as several individuals with expertise in various areas working in serial fashion, separate from each other. Although overall objectives may be similar, they rarely work or meet together and even less frequently interact with the intent to overlap and interweave skill sets and care plans to arrive at those objectives. The multidisciplinary team is characterized by clear role definitions and consistent maintenance (even guarding) of the boundaries among those roles. A sports analogy would be a football or baseball team where each player has a specific position and assignment with only occasional deviation from these roles. Decision making and authority are centralized by design, and there is little, if any, tolerance, let alone permission, for innovation.

The interdisciplinary group may be composed of identical professional members as the multidisciplinary paradigm, but the role definitions are purposefully blurred and the boundaries are widely overlapping. Authority is shared, as is decision making, and innovation is encouraged wherever necessitated by patient need and circumstance. Referring to the previous sports analogy, the interdisciplinary group functions more like a basketball or soccer team where success results from fluid and spontaneous innovation, with some set plays but ample flexibility to adapt to the demands of changing situations. Roles are expected to be shared or traded as needed. In order to achieve this level of fluid teamwork, a high level of communication must be maintained, which requires considerable maturity, trust, and intimacy. These professional expectations may exceed those required in other, less-interdependent healthcare environments.

Such teams or groups require an unusual degree of attention to interpersonal relationships in order to maintain the necessary level of mutual trust and understanding of one another's strengths and limitations. This need exposes the team to a significant risk, however. In order to achieve and sustain the ideal level of professional intimacy, it is often necessary to engage in a level of sharing that feels more personal than professional to the team members. As a result, team members may begin to look to the team to meet their personal needs and even to resolve issues in their personal lives. This is the one boundary a team must not cross. To do so runs the risk of undermining the team's professional functioning and blurs the focus of the team: delivering the highest quality of care possible to patients and families in need.

To maintain an optimal functional level, team members often must share and explore emotional reactions their patients and families trigger in them. However, this sort of sharing and self-examination should always be undertaken to further their professional functions, not as a means of meeting personal needs. Those must be met outside of the work environment in the intimacy of one's own personal life or in one's own decisions to partake of professional help in sorting through difficult emotional experiences.

A high-functioning team must be flexible enough to reconfigure itself in response to the needs of each patient and family. This requires mature professionals who are able to deal with the personal and strong emotional issues hospice work engenders: one's own mortality, the motivations and sources that compel us to be a caretaker, one's need to be liked, ability to tolerate patients' anger, and so many others. While there can be intense and challenging issues, they should always and only be addressed in the effort to further the work at hand. We come together to assess and plan for the care of our patients and their families, not to address our own needs. This point cannot be overstated: the focus must always be what serves the patient's and family's needs. The valuable time of team meetings needs to be spent understanding and addressing patient care issues first, then professional and administrative issues as necessary in order to fulfill care plans, and finally, those issues that arise between or among team members that are an impediment to care delivery. To depart from this healthy and functional approach is to depart from the reason the team exists.

The Structured Team Meeting

IDT Care Conference Format

This is a guide only, and it should be "molded" to fit the needs and unique circumstances of each team and the patients/families under care. Adherence to the *basic* format will ensure that most key issues are addressed and a focus on all pertinent elements is maintained. Keeping this format in mind during patient visits will also help to organize thinking and prioritize care issues.

Recommended IDT Conference Format for Patient Care Managers

- All disciplines represented and signed in
- Deaths reviewed since last IDT conference; lessons learned, thoughts and feelings about the care given and dying process
- New admissions in home and other residential care locations (nursing home, long-term care, assisted living) and inpatient settings
- Review patients who have been recertified since the last team meeting and review/schedule physician or nurse practitioner visits for those patients in need of a face-to-face visit (for recertification of hospice eligibility in benefit periods 3 and beyond) in the next 30 days. Regulations regarding hospice eligibility and recertification have evolved and will likely continue to do so. It is imperative that your Director of Compliance be involved in certification/recertification processes and related documentation requirements so that your program is not vulnerable to loss of revenue due to technical denials.
- Review of caseload
  - Plan of care is effective and should continue
  - Plan of care needs to be modified based on changes in biomedical, psychosocial, spiritual, practical issues
    - Indications for continuous care, inpatient admission (general inpatient and respite)
    - "Two-minute" case presentation by designated case manager, including patient name, age, gender, referring/primary physician, terminal diagnosis (*note: as much of this type of rostering that can be prepared in advance and automated, by using electronic media and projecting for the entire IDT to see, the better, because this will save time and reduce paper*), care situation (home, other), primary caregivers, current medications
      - Coexisting medical problems—Is there an adequate "database"? Is there a need for more information?
      - Interval history since last presentation
      - Symptoms well managed? Goals/needs met?
      - If symptoms are not well controlled, propose most likely etiology and specific treatment plan
      - Continued problems, issues, needs, etc.
      - New problems, issues, needs, etc.
      - Progression of disease or level of debility (e.g., weight loss, decreased appetite, decreased energy/activity/function/ADLs, etc.); add specifics to documentation

- Review of determinants of limited prognosis for hospice admission diagnosis (supporting documents in medical record?)
- Summary of hospice end outcomes: five "quality of life" domains as they pertain to the ongoing care of the patient/family under review—
  - Physical symptoms (pain, nausea, etc.)
  - Physical functions (activity, etc.)
  - Intrapersonal dimension (emotional status, self-view, etc.)
  - Interpersonal status (relationships, communication, conflicts, etc.)
  - Transcendent issues (issues of "meaning," existence, spiritual matters, etc.)—

  in relation to the major end outcomes of end-of-life care:
  - Safe and comfortable dying
  - Self-determined life closure
  - Effective coping with loss and grief
  - Communication with referring physician: when, how, what?
  - Is communication profile on referring physician complete (i.e., profile of type of communication [telephone call, fax, email, letter] by whom and how often preferred by referring/primary care physician)?
- The plan of care should be derived from the above, including plan for communication with referring physician, delegation of duties to specific IDT members (who, what, when, how often, goals), and next scheduled review by IDT
- A 15- to 20-minute mini "inservice" by team member(s) selected the previous week regarding a topic that emerged as "begging" deeper understanding and discussion by the team, or identified by patient care manager, such as symptom management, assessment/diagnosis, psychosocial issues, spiritual care issues, process/system (documentation, regulatory, compliance, etc.), bereavement
- Identification of topic and discussion leaders for next week's IDT conference "inservice"

Addressing Needs over Time

This section is meant as a guide for helping patients, families, and the caregiving team understand the dynamics of the last phase of life. Timeframes represent generalizations that will need to be tailored to pertain to specific cases, but overall, they should help orchestrate care and prepare for the changes that tend to occur with advanced illness no matter where the patient resides.

Professional caregiver responsibilities, duties, and levels of involvement are assigned to those disciplines (core members of the IDT) that are most likely to have the greatest expertise in attending to the specified functions and needs of patients during the various phases of disease progression. These are not meant to be exclusive by any means. The true strength of the IDT is the ability of its core and additional members (e.g., pharmacists, nutritionists, functional restoration therapists), regardless of specific discipline, to fulfill multiple roles as the situation dictates, limited only by professional practice licensure restrictions and the experience and proven ability of the individual.

Hospice IDT Members: Approximately 6 Months or Longer Before Death

Patient and Family

- Patients are usually coherent and able to walk. They may have symptoms from previous medical treatments.
- Patient and family exhibit initial stages of grief with feelings of potential loss, anger, and denial.
- There may be humor and a heightened sense of living, all very appropriate.
- Some symptoms of decline (weight loss, fatigue) and a sense of the seriousness of the illness usually emerge.
- Initial signs of stress, with symptoms of depression, anxiety, or fear, should be anticipated and discussed.
- Family members wonder how they will cope.

Physician

- Reviews medical history; examines patient when indicated and certifies for hospice care
- Works with IDT to develop plan of care and authorizes medical orders
- Manages pain and other distressing symptoms
- Hospice physician attends interdisciplinary team meetings and confers with attending/referring physician as needed

RN/Case Manager

- Communicates with physician, family, and patient to develop initial plan of care
- Ensures that medical orders and durable medical equipment are in place and trains/instructs nonprofessional caregivers
- Coordinates plan of care, provides direct patient care, and directs other nurses, aides, and volunteers
- Manages resources
- Establishes rapport and trust with patient, family, and attending physician
- Furthers discussions about advance care plans and end-of-life decisions
- Coordinates input at interdisciplinary team conferences

CNA/HHA

- Initiates personal care program under direction of RN case manager
- Establishes rapport with patient and family and provides personal care
- Conferences with case manager in developing care instructions

Social Worker

- Elaborates hospice philosophy and services
- Assesses patient and family needs from a psychosocial and spiritual perspective
- Collaborates in development of a plan of care according to needs, goals, preferences, and hopes

- Provides support, problem solving, coping strategies, and connections to other community resources as needed

Chaplain

- Collaborates with other team members as care plan is developed
- Meets with patient and/or family at their request for spiritual or related care
- Helps other team members providing psychosocial support and dealing with difficult issues

Volunteer

- Volunteer manager collaborates with interdisciplinary team to determine patient/family needs that may be fulfilled by volunteers
- Arranges visits or telephone calls according to patient and family wishes and needs
- Assists with respite breaks and provides volunteer companionship when needed

Hospice IDT Members: A Few Months Before Death

Patient and Family

- Patient has decreased appetite, fatigue, and weight loss.
- Physical signs and symptoms are more evident. Family begins to reconcile feelings and plan for imminent death.
- Patient begins to accept the fact that disease is incurable and time is limited.
- Physical decline is apparent, and increased attention is spent on coping with progressive pain and other symptoms.
- Patient may show signs of social withdrawal, and the family may show signs of stress from caregiving and anticipatory grief.

Physician

- Works with IDT to evaluate symptoms, manage pain, and contribute to plan of care, adjusting medical orders as necessary
- Evaluates for continued hospice eligibility per guidelines

RN/Case Manager

- Monitors implementation of care plan with increasing attention to symptom management
- Assists IDT in evaluating and managing psychosocial needs

CNA/HHA

- Provides or assists in personal care as needed and directed
- Offers companionship
- Provides feedback to IDT about unmet needs and changes in status

Social Worker

- Monitors psychosocial plan of care and adapts it to changing needs and circumstances as they unfold

- Provides ongoing assessment of patient's and family's adjustment to the illness and impending loss and helps determine timing of respite based upon coping abilities
- Provides ongoing emotional support

Chaplain

- Provides spiritual and emotional support and counseling
- Communicates with clergy or lay spiritual leader of family/patient choosing
- Encourages and helps arrange rituals that offer meaning and support to the patient/family

Volunteer

- Works with volunteer coordinator, IDT, and patient/family to be aware of unspoken emotional or practical needs
- Spends "unstructured" time with patient and family in order to allow free exchange of concerns and feelings
- Helps relieve boredom for patient by engaging in whatever activities are feasible
- Works with IDT to identify ways and means to relieve caregiving burden

Hospice IDT Members: Last Few Weeks and Days

Patient and Family

- Symptoms tend to increase, with control of pain and shortness of breath chief symptom relief concerns.
- Fatigue becomes a dominant feature and the patient may be bedridden, requiring intensification of personal care and prevention of skin breakdown.
- The patient may alternately be extremely demanding and very withdrawn.
- Reinitiation of discussion regarding signs of imminent death, dealing with terminal care issues and funeral arrangements, is usually desired.

Physician

- Works with IDT to review symptoms with a focus on pain and other distressing symptom relief
- Contributes to biomedical aspects of the plan of care, adjusting medical orders as necessary
- Visits patient and family if symptoms are not readily controlled
- Available for rapid adjustment in medication orders and route of drug delivery as conditions dictate

RN/Case Manager

- Monitors patient closely, with increased frequency of home visits as dictated by changing conditions
- Frequent review of symptom control
- Coordinates care by members of IDT to support family and manage terminal care needs
- Determines whether continuous care or inpatient care is needed
- Instructs family in signs of imminent dying and to call so that attendance at death, or immediately thereafter, is possible

CNA/HHA

- Responds to changes in plan of care as directed by case manager
- Special attention to oral care, perineum, and pressure points
- Identifies special needs to IDT

Social Worker

- Anticipates and assesses for heightened anxiety and emotional distress, as well as caregiver fatigue
- Assists patient and family in resolving conflicts and making closure, expressing thoughts and feelings
- Helps family with funeral planning

Chaplain

- Continues to provide spiritual and emotional support
- Provides pastoral care as requested by the patient and family
- May assist with funeral arrangements and rituals
- Helps prepare family and patient for separation, and looks for ways to help heal relationships that are stressed, facilitating closure and the final opportunity for personal growth before death
- Familiarizes family with bereavement program, especially if bereavement counselor is a different person

Hospice IDT Members: After Death

Family

- Family experiencing loss and grief

Physician

- May communicate with family; may send condolence note

RN/Case Manager

- Calls or visits family
- May attend funeral
- Assists bereavement counselor in assessing family's bereavement needs
- Completes documentation

CNA/HHA

- May attend funeral or visit family

Social Worker

- Calls or visits family
- May attend funeral
- Assesses family for signs of dysfunctional grieving and other psychosocial problems
- Makes referrals to appropriate resources

Chaplain/Bereavement

- May call or visit family
- May attend funeral
- Instructs family about grief recovery and support groups

Counselor

- Provides bereavement counseling as needed
- Plans and implements memorial services
- Directs staff and volunteers to maintain contact with family at regular intervals for 13 months

Volunteer

- May call or visit family
- May attend funeral
- Bereavement volunteers offer support for 13 months.

Documentation

The Clinical Documentation Process Serves Several Important Functions

- It is the structure that describes what is to be done, what has been done, and what has been accomplished to meet the patient's/family's goals.
- It is the continuous and memorialized record of the patient and his or her experiences through hospice.
- Well-constructed records provide unambiguous and clear communication among all hospice care staff.
- The medical record is the means by which reimbursement for services is justified and determined.

Documents Must Serve the Needs of Many Different Persons and Organizations

Patient/Family

- Informative documents, brief and to the point
- As few signatures as possible
- Confidentiality
- Pertinent information only (respect for privacy, dignity, ethical boundaries) for delivery of quality care

Attending Physician and Referral Sources

- Brief, complete, summarized information
- Minimal paperwork burden

Interdisciplinary Team and Administrative Personnel

- Legible and timely entries
- Access to information
- Complete information
- Logical flow of information

Clinical Facilities (e.g., hospital, nursing home, inpatient unit)

- Facilitate continuity of care
- Logical flow of plan of care

- Summary information, encapsulated to provide brief but complete picture of the patient and other pertinent facts at time of admission

Regulatory Agencies, Third-Party Payers, Accreditation Entities

- Proof of eligibility
- Zero tolerance for fraud/abuse of public funds
- Required for payment
- Critical step in regulatory compliance
- Complete entries
- Signed entries
- Adequate narrative to "tell the story" or "paint a picture" of the patient's/family's circumstances and experience through hospice
- Processes of care (evaluations, plans of care, interventions)
- Outcomes of care

Documentation and Risk Management

- Use full signature; date and time all entries.
- Complete all medical records and documentation forms (i.e., fill in the blanks).
- Be specific; elaborate only as necessary.
- Individual viewpoints are reviewed and reconciled at IDT conference, not in the written record. Discussions and challenge of ideas/perspectives are appropriate and welcome at IDT conference but have no place in the medical record.
- Report adverse occurrences/mistakes on incident reports.
- Legibility is key; with the advent of electronic health records (EHR) there are fewer handwritten notes, but if there are, they need to be readable.
- Use only universally accepted abbreviations; when in doubt, spell it out.
- Read back verbal orders and note this confirmation to reduce medication errors.

Documentation Needs Specific to Hospice Care

- Routine home care: records must tell the story of the patient and reflect the patterns of care and the hospice experience.
- General inpatient care: records must clearly show the indications for a change in level of care.
  - Symptoms out of control
  - Efforts to regain control in the home
  - What interventions can be done in the inpatient setting that cannot be done at home?
  - Caregiver or environmental crisis needs to be well described.
  - If death is imminent, describe findings in detail.
  - Daily assessments, care plan, and IDT involvement need to be documented.
  - All interventions must be charted in detail, taking nothing for granted.
  - Specify what comfort measures were provided.

- Must have frequent documentation (i.e., every 1 to 2 hours), not a synopsis; no "block charting" (e.g., 1–4 a.m.); charting must include specific times and events
- Document what the medical crisis was and continues to be that justifies this level of care.
- Initial certification and recertification: supply ample narrative that describes clinical parameters with respect to the hospice diagnosis and ongoing trajectory toward death.
- Define as clearly as possible "related" and "unrelated" conditions and therapies in relation to hospice diagnosis (e.g., diuretics are related to the diagnosis of end-stage heart failure, whereas insulin would be unrelated to this diagnosis).
- Utilize prognostic worksheets and guidelines and supplement with observations that support a prognosis of limited life expectancy.
  - Track objective measures of decline (weight loss, reduced appetite, decreasing functional abilities, etc.).
  - When decline is not apparent, describe care that may be leading to functional improvement and plans to review prognosis if improvement in status is sustained.
- Home health aide/certified nurse assistant supervisory visits: document supervision every 2 weeks—ensure compliance with state regulations.
- IDT communication: comprehensive care plan updates are essential.
  - Summarize communications in easy-to-review form.
  - Clearly state who (include discipline), what, when, why, anticipated goals, contingency plans, and next evaluation.
- Nursing home documentation: the record must show an integrated plan of care that clearly and specifically delineates hospice functions and identifies responsible staff:
  - All care must be documented.
  - Nursing home chart must have a specific place for hospice records.
  - Medical orders must be duplicated and integrated into comprehensive plan of care.

Accountability

- All hospice staff are individually responsible and accountable for completing their respective portion(s) of the medical record in a legible and timely manner—this is a fundamental expectation and there are no exceptions.
- The RN case manager is chiefly responsible and accountable for coordinating care and ensuring completeness of the medical records of the patients he or she is managing and, in turn, will monitor others' compliance. If deficiencies are not immediately corrected, the program director, or equivalent position, is to be notified so that corrective actions can be taken.

Section 2

Personal, Social, and Environmental Processes

Abuse in the Home

SITUATION: Domestic abuse, neglect, or exploitation interfering with end-of-life care

Findings

- Physical evidence of abuse/neglect/exploitation
- Expression of ambivalent feelings of anger, jealousy, hurt, fear, sadness, guilt, self-righteousness, apologies, promises, or martyrdom
- Use of intimidation and manipulation as a way to maintain control and avoid feelings or generate personal gains
- Family history of verbal, emotional, physical, economic, or sexual abuse
- Use of defense mechanisms: minimization, justification, denial, and blame
- Depression, suicidal ideation

Assessment

Physical

- Environmental or corporeal evidence of abuse, neglect, violence

Psychosocial

- Patient as victim of abuse. NOTE: If abuse and/or neglect is suspected by a mandated reporter, this necessitates a referral to Adult Protective Services (APS). Adult Protective Services is not equipped, nor is it meant, for emergency response. IN CASE OF IMMINENT DANGER, LAW ENFORCEMENT MUST BE CONTACTED IMMEDIATELY. An APS referral, if disclosed to patient and/or caregiver, can be framed in such a way as to indicate additional support for patient and/or caregiver.
  - Identify patient/caregiver's perception of situation.
  - Assess history of abuse/neglect.
  - Assess patient fears.
  - Identify present threats of harm.
  - Identify if caregiver insists on staying close and speaking for patient.
  - Assess if patient is reluctant to speak or disagree in presence of caregiver.
  - Identify symptoms of depression, panic attacks, substance abuse, feelings of isolation, and post-traumatic stress reactions.
  - Determine patient/caregiver resources to address issue.
  - Determine support systems available.

- Identify caregiver's ambivalent feelings/desire for revenge as barrier to providing adequate patient care.
- Assess for risk of suicide.
- Patient as abuser
  - Identify patient/caregiver's perception of situation.
    - Assess safety if patient is still physically capable of abuse.
    - Identify verbal and emotional abuse to caregiver by patient.
    - Assess need for control, manipulation, intimidation.
    - Assess presence of denial, minimization, justification, and blame as defense mechanisms.
    - Assess for intense emotional reaction to loss, including suicide potential.

Processes of Care

Psychosocial

- Patient as victim of abuse
  - Facilitate discussion of perceptions and feelings.
  - Acknowledge and encourage use of previously effective coping skills.
  - Assist patient/caregiver in accepting limits imposed by illness.
  - Provide education on safety issues.
  - See patient alone when possible.
  - Visit with two staff members, one to see caregiver and one to see patient, to obtain clear information.
  - Monitor willingness/ability to comply with treatment plan.
  - Consider transfer to alternative location (e.g., care facility) if need arises.
  - Confer with team members regarding intervention plan and options for care.
- Patient as abuser
  - Provide education on safety issues.
  - Develop safety plan with team and caregiver.
  - Assist in setting limits and provide clear communication about unacceptable behaviors to patient.
  - Encourage patient to identify feelings underneath anger (e.g., does patient feel a need for control? This may not be the only feeling present).
  - Support caregiver in taking care of own needs.
  - Explore possibility of providing additional support to give caregiver respite (respite care, volunteers).
  - Discuss alternatives with caregiver in situations of high risk/burnout (e.g., care facility placement).
  - Confer with bereavement support staff regarding high risk for dysfunctional grief.

Goals/Outcomes

- Patient/caregiver will show improved ability to cope.
- Patient/caregiver/hospice staff will be aware of need for clear limits/boundaries for safety.
- Patient/caregiver will identify strategies to address needs in the terminal situation.
- Decreased incidence of domestic abuse/violence/neglect

Documentation in the Medical Record

Initial and Ongoing Physical Assessment

• Examination findings suggestive of abuse, neglect

Initial and Ongoing Psychosocial Assessment

• Areas of abuse, neglect, and violence as identified by patient, family, and staff

Interdisciplinary Progress Notes and IDT Care Plan

• Specific interventions to assist patient/caregiver
• Patient/caregiver response to intervention
• Ongoing evaluation

Advance Care Planning and Directives for Health-Care Interventions

SITUATION: Patient has preferences about medical interventions and chooses to protect his/her rights by specifying the type of medical care desired.

Findings

• Patient wants to make decisions and protect his/her rights.
• Patient wants to clarify preferences to physician and caregiver/family.
• Family has differing ideas about treatment for patient.
• Patient wants to communicate choices while still able.

Assessment

Psychosocial

• Assess if advance directives have been previously completed.
• Assess patient/caregiver's awareness/understanding of value/purpose of advance directives.
• Assess patient's desire to complete forms with or without assistance from hospice staff.

Processes of Care

Psychosocial

• Educate patient and family about different types of advance directives and processes:
  • Power of Attorney: Patient gives power to transact business on his/her behalf when he/she cannot do so because of time or distance (although physically able).
  • Durable Power of Attorney: Patient gives power to transact business on his/her behalf when patient is no longer physically or mentally able.
  • Living Will: This is an advance directive that states what types of care or medical interventions patient prefers or wishes to avoid under various circumstances.

- Durable Power of Attorney for Health Care: This legal document protects patient-care choices by naming an advocate who makes decisions on behalf of patient when a physician determines the patient does not have capacity to make his/her own medical decisions. The process for determining incapacity varies by state; providers should be aware of the regulations in every jurisdiction in which they practice.
- Do Not (Attempt to) Resuscitate: This directive states that the patient refuses certain *potentially* life-prolonging medical interventions, such as cardiopulmonary resuscitation, chest compressions, endotracheal intubation, and defibrillation.
- Physician Orders for Life-Sustaining Treatment (POLST): The National POLST Paradigm is an approach to end-of-life planning based on conversations between patients, loved ones, and health-care professionals designed to ensure that seriously ill or frail patients can choose the treatments they want or do not want and that their wishes are documented and honored. (Quoted directly from http://www.polst.org/. Last accessed April 19, 2016.)
- The acronyms used by states adhering to the POLST paradigm vary, with POST (Physician Orders for Scope of Treatment), MOST (Medical Orders for Scope of Treatment), and MOLST (Medical Orders for Life-Sustaining Treatment) being the most common. More information can be obtained from http://www.polst.org/ (accessed April, 2016).
- Guardianship: Parent is the guardian for minor child unless a legal action rules otherwise. Court-appointed guardianship by petition can be temporary, financial, or custodial.
- Facilitate discussion regarding choices for treatment/care with family when patient is no longer able to participate in these decisions.
- Facilitate discussion with patient/caregiver regarding appropriate advance directives and choice of advocate.
- Assist patient in completing advance directives form/document.
- Procure a copy of advance directive for patient record.

Goals/Outcomes

- Patient will voice preferences about current and future medical care and actions to be taken in the event of loss of decision-making ability.
- Caregiver/family/advocate will have clear directions for understanding patient choices.
- Minimize ambiguity and ambivalence in all parties.
- Completion of life in a manner and setting consistent with wishes and values (i.e., "self-determined life closure")

Documentation in the Medical Record

Initial Psychosocial Assessment

- Need for advance directives as identified by patient/caregiver/social work/admission team
- Options discussed
- Forms/documents completed
- Copy of advance directives and documents in medical record

Interdisciplinary Progress Notes

- Documentation of processes of advance care planning that have been completed

IDT Care Plan

- Plan for carrying out processes of advance care planning

Changes in Body Image and Loss of Independence

SITUATION: Patient's/caregiver's reactions to changes in body image and loss of independence associated with advanced illness are causing distress and difficulty coping/functioning.

Findings

- Persistent, preoccupying, and intense expressions of anger, frustration, loneliness, loss of self-esteem, embarrassment, shame, guilt, etc. due to altered physical appearance, altered functional ability, changes in social/family identity/status
- Avoidance of discussion regarding appearance
- Loss of functional abilities due to disease process
- Increasing dependence upon others for care
- Caregiver loss of previously relied upon companion support; change in roles
- Social isolation
- Self-imposed disengagement from feelings, family members, friends, outside community
- Pronounced depression
- Sexual dysfunction
- Suicidal thoughts

Assessment

Biomedical

- Identify disease-related, postsurgical, or postradiation alterations in external physical features or means to communicate (e.g., amputation [including mastectomy; orchiectomy]; ostomies; open sores/wounds/lesions; scars or other disfigurement; vocal/visual/auditory impairment)

Psychosocial/Spiritual

- Identify primary issue(s) of concern.
- Explore patient/caregiver perception of body image, value of appearance, functional limitations.
- Determine patient/caregiver capacity to address the issues.
- Determine support systems available and nature/basis of faith/beliefs.
- Identify who patient will allow to help provide care.
- Assess for history of suicidal ideation or behavior.
- Rule out other confounding issues/comorbidities (e.g., depression, anxiety disorder, agoraphobia).
- Identify history/style of coping.

- Assess impact of illness/appearance upon sexuality.
- Assess financial resources available for supplementary help if needed.

Processes of Care

Biomedical

- Treat identified mood disorder with pharmacotherapy if indicated, per severity and diagnostic criteria.
- Ensure that expert-level attention to wound and ostomy care, prosthetics, and other restorative or rehabilitative therapies, appropriate to the patient's overall circumstances, is arranged.

Psychosocial/Spiritual

- Facilitate expressions of feelings and perceptions; acknowledge losses.
- Address real versus perceived body image and functional limitations.
- Acknowledge and encourage use of previously effective coping skills.
- Provide information regarding progression of illness.
- Assist patient/caregiver to develop new coping skills for positive self-image.
- Encourage patient/caregiver participation in support groups.
- Treat identified mood disorder/phobic behavior with counseling.
- If symptoms are not responding to basic counseling approaches, assist in providing resources/referral to treat mood disorder/phobic behavior and support patient/family through crisis periods.
- Assist patient in finding meaning in past achievements through life review.

Practical

- Obtain consultation or access resources for use of prostheses, wigs, cosmetics, etc.
- Facilitate placement for respite and/or residential care if needed.

Goals/Outcomes

- Condition-specific optimal physical and communicative capacities.
- Patient/caregiver will demonstrate or verbalize improved coping ability.
- Patient/caregiver will express higher level of acceptance of alterations in body image and changes in functional abilities.
- Patient will exhibit fewer signs/symptoms of depression, anxiety, phobic behavior.
- Patient will feel less isolated.

Documentation in the Medical Record

Initial and Ongoing Physical Assessment

- Relevant physical findings and changes over time

Initial Psychosocial Assessment

- Evidence of poor body image/dependency and inadequate coping

Interdisciplinary Progress Notes

- Manifestations of changes in body image and loss of independence
- Ongoing assessments and results of interventions

IDT Care Plan
• Defined interventions and expected outcomes

Changes in Family Dynamics

SITUATION: Family dynamics are having a negative impact upon effective end-of-life care.

Findings

• Family member(s) report high level of stress due to inability to cope effectively with crisis of impending death and eventual loss of patient.
• Family member(s) exhibit difficulty with intimacy (dependency, conflict, or detachment).
• Family member(s) express concern/confusion about changes in roles, duties, lifestyle, and family interaction patterns.
• Family member(s) report other existing stressful issues requiring time and attention.

Assessment

Psychosocial/Spiritual

• Outline a "family tree" that describes the family system and defines roles, expectations, relationships, and issues.
• Identify family interaction patterns (e.g., close, conflicted, enmeshed, distant, or estranged).
• Ask family member(s) to describe their perception of family in the context of the patient's terminal illness.
• Identify previous experiences and patterns of dealing with loss individually and as a family system.
• Assess appearance of harmony or disharmony among various family members.
• Assess impact of conflicts on care of patient.
• Assess position the patient maintains within the family structure.
• Assess ability of family to communicate about dying.
• Assess existence of self-destructive/family-impacting behaviors (e.g., substance abuse, gambling or other addictive disorders) with any immediate family members, including the patient.
• Assess history of mental illness, abuse, or antisocial behavior.
• Assess factors of illiteracy, or mental and physical limitations.
• Assess experiences and attitudes of family in dealing with the medical community or with authority figures.
• Assess willingness and ability to understand and utilize instructions and interventions.
• Assess impact of ethnic/cultural background, values, beliefs, attitudes, and family rituals/traditions.
• Assess ability of family system to access internal and external resources.

Processes of Care

Psychosocial/Spiritual

- Facilitate discussion of useful strengths and resources that helped family member(s) in previous crises (e.g., cohesion, concern for each other, commitment to family, pride, loyalty, utilization of external resources).
- Increase awareness of family rules, boundaries, patterns of communications, and role expectations.
- Encourage dialogue and expressions of feelings about illness and dying, when appropriate.
- Identify role-change strain/conflict and assist in redistribution of roles and responsibilities.
- Assist family member(s) in setting short-, intermediate-, and long-term goals and acknowledge progress made in achieving them.
- Facilitate discussion of previous or ongoing hurt feelings that have potential for resolution/healing.
- Facilitate referral to external resources as needed.
- Facilitate arrangements for respite care, if appropriate and available, in family with high level of stress.
- Assist family in shared life review and reminiscence, if appropriate.
- Assist family in the task of preparing for the death of a family member.
- Assist family in the task of beginning to prepare for life after the death of the family member.
- Assist family in having realistic expectations of hospice care.
- Provide emotional support to family.
- Address resistance to psychosocial interventions.
- Develop plan of care with patient, family, and interdisciplinary team and continue to monitor progress.
- Facilitate family conference.

Goals/Outcomes

- Family shows increased ability to cope with the imminent death of a family member in the context of the family system.
- Family feels reduction in levels of stress.
- Family will have strengthened external/internal resources to care for patient at home, if this is the most appropriate setting.
- Family will have increased ability to process grief reactions following death of loved one.

Documentation in the Medical Record

Initial Psychosocial/Spiritual Assessment

- Dynamics of family system affecting care of terminally ill patient

Interdisciplinary Progress Notes

- Summary of IDT conferences related to family dynamics affecting care
- Results of interventions
- Summary of ongoing evaluations

IDT Care Plan

- Resources and problem-solving skills to be relayed/taught/recommended
- Social work interventions: who, what, when, how often; and specify goals
- Chaplain interventions: who, what, when, how often; and specify goals

Completing Worldly Business and Life Closure

SITUATION: Patient has a need to complete certain tasks before death.

Findings

- Patient expressing lack of completion in worldly affairs
- Patient/caregiver expressing desire for completion with relationships
- Patient expressing "weariness" with life; lack of purpose/meaning in living
- Patient/caregiver unable to accept patient's death
- Patient/caregiver unable to resolve spiritual issues
- Patient/caregiver working toward balance of body, mind, and spirit in the face of death

Assessment

Psychosocial/Spiritual

- Identify patient/caregiver perception of situation.
- Identify patient/caregiver capacity to address life closure and/or unresolved issues.
- Review past life experiences, changes in roles, losses, and previously effective coping skills.
- Identify role-change strain/conflict.
- Identify patient/caregiver experiences, concerns, and fears regarding the dying process.
- Assess need for spiritual care and anticipatory grief support.
- Assess patient/caregiver perception of current quality of life and future concerns.

Processes of Care

Psychosocial/Spiritual

Worldly Affairs

- Support patient/caregiver in settling financial affairs and making final arrangements.
- Link patient/caregiver with appropriate resources: financial/estate planner, viatical settlement organizations, legal counsel, etc.
- Facilitate patient's writing of an estate will.

Meaning and Purpose in Life

- Assist patient in coming to terms with personal and existential loss represented by one's dying.

- Facilitate patient/caregiver expressed need to search for meaning in the dying experience.
- Review past life experiences, role changes, and losses.
- Reinforce previously effective coping skills.
- Help patient/caregiver search the meaning and depth of his or her particular faith/beliefs.
- Assist patient in acceptance of dependence/loss of independence.
- Refer to "complementary" therapies: music, art, massage, etc.
- Assist patient toward growth/development in the context of personal grieving, loss, and suffering.

Relationships

- Present grief as a unique opportunity to address and heal unresolved issues and fears.
- Facilitate closure with important relationships by expressing sorrow, forgiveness, affection, love, gratitude, and appreciation, and saying "goodbye."
- Assist patient in expressing self-worth and forgiveness.
- Involve caregiver in planning for emotional, spiritual, psychosocial, and physical needs and facilitate implementation.
- Facilitate discussion of useful strengths and resources that helped family members in previous crises.
- Identify role-change strain/conflict and assist in redistribution of roles/responsibilities.
- Assist family in the task of preparing for the death of the patient.
- Facilitate and validate family rituals.
- Assist family in the task of beginning to prepare for life after the death of the patient.
- Refer, as appropriate, to grief support counselor for anticipatory grief.

Dying

- Respond to questions and concerns about the signs and symptoms indicating patient is approaching death.
- Explore patient/caregiver experiences, concerns, and fears regarding dying process.
- Support patient in moving from a transient world to whatever his/her sense of the transcendent may be.

Spiritual Issues

- Explore issues of guilt and human and/or divine forgiveness.
- Encourage spiritual practices of meditation; engagement with music, poetry, literature, nature, or science; keeping a written journal or audio/visual tape, imagery, prayers, and/or spiritual/religious rites.
- Explore belief, faith, and trust in higher dimension that provide patient/caregiver support.
- Assess need for spiritual care.
- Respond to specific pastoral requests.

- Encourage emotional/spiritual sharing among patient/family members.
- Facilitate patient/caregiver connection with his or her preferred religious institution, if any.

Goals/Outcomes

- Patient/caregiver will express increased sense of completion in worldly affairs.
- Patient/caregiver will express increased sense of meaning and purpose.
- Patient/caregiver will express increased sense of completion with relationships.
- Patient/caregiver is able to express acceptance of his/her death if possible.
- Patient/caregiver will feel that there has been resolution of spiritual issues.
- Patient/caregiver will have a sense of personal completion to life.

Documentation in the Medical Record

Initial Psychosocial/Spiritual Assessment

- Major emotional, psychosocial, and spiritual issues of concern identified by patient, family, and hospice staff
- Coping skills, resources, preferences identified

Interdisciplinary Progress Note

- Continued identification of issues as per initial assessment
- Ongoing identification of goals
- Results and goals/outcomes summarized

IDT Care Plan

- Interventions planned by staff (who, what, when, frequency, goals)
- Plans for ongoing evaluation

Controlled Substances: Misuse and Abuse

SITUATION: Medically inappropriate use of controlled substances in the home is having a negative impact on end-of-life care.

Findings

- Pattern of unexplained disappearance of medications
- Consistent shortage of prescribed controlled substance without appropriate communication to care team about medical necessity to change dose or schedule
- History or evidence of substance use among patient, family, and friends
- Deliberate guarding or expression of need to guard medications from others
- Environmental clues that suggest drug diversion
- Unusual patient or family perceptions of symptom management

Assessment

Psychosocial/Spiritual

- Identify substance abuse as reported by patient/caregiver and/or observed by professional care team member(s).
- Identify characteristics of chemically dependent family system as evidenced by the following patterns:
  - Denial
  - Control
  - Conflict
  - Distrust
  - Unresolved losses
  - Secrets
  - Resistance to outsiders
  - Blaming
  - Domestic chaos
  - Violence
  - Falsification
- Identify prior or current use of formal treatment and support programs (i.e., AA, NA, Al-Anon, Nar-Anon, etc.).
- Understand patient and family perceptions regarding symptom management and substance abuse.
- Assess impact of substance use on ability to provide patient care or to cope with dying.
- Refer to the *Diagnostic & Statistical Manual, Fifth Edition (DSM-5)* for information about Substance Abuse Disorders.
- Assess need to intervene and/or refer to specialty counseling or mental health services based on impact of substance abuse.
- Understand special social/cultural/ethnic/religious perspectives (rituals) of patient/caregiver/family member(s) on controlled substance use.

Processes of Care

Educational

- Provide information regarding effects of substance abuse on physical symptoms and grief processes.
- Provide information and instruction regarding achievable expectations regarding symptom management.

Psychosocial/Spiritual

- Explore motivations for substance use (abuse), especially if a new problem:
  - Depression/despair/hopelessness
  - Anxiety
  - Fear
  - Anticipated grief
  - Other conflicts
- Involve family in talking about options and interventions.
- Notify prescribing professional health-care providers (physicians, nurse practitioners, physician assistants).

- Use appropriate referral sources.
- Develop unified team approach.

Practical/Procedural

- Schedule II/III medicines (e.g., opioids, benzodiazepines) are to be reordered by only one prescriber or nurse manager.
- Consider using a formal "Treatment Agreement" (sometimes referred to as a "Treatment Contract"), co-signed by all prescribing physicians/clinicians and members of the IDT.
- Renew only one-week supply at a time.
- Count medication carefully each nursing visit.
- Implement measures to secure medications in the home (safe storage).
- Consider discussing or implementing urine drug testing if contextually appropriate and useful as a management tool.
- Review safe disposal procedures.

Goals/Outcomes

- Patient/caregiver will verbalize understanding of appropriate medical use of prescription medications for symptom management (schedule and dose).
- Patient/family will utilize outside resources for specific issues related to substance abuse as necessary to attain patient end-of-life goals.
- Effect(s) of substance abuse on patient care or ability to cope will be minimized.

Documentation in the Medical Record

Initial Psychosocial/Spiritual Assessment

- Explicit findings of substance abuse/drug diversion
- Current and projected impact on patient/caregiver/family

Interdisciplinary Progress Note

- Interventions carried out (who, what, when)
- Expected goals/outcomes
- Results of interventions
- Findings of ongoing evaluations and assessments

IDT Care Plan

- Schedule of interventions
- Contingency plans if interventions do not achieve hoped-for outcomes
- Schedule of follow-up and reevaluations
- Changes in care plan with justification

Cultural Differences: Respect, Understanding, and Adapting Care

NOTE: The citizenry of the United States is ethnically, religiously, and racially diverse. This brief overview is meant to serve as both a reminder and a guide so that professional caregivers can meet the varied needs of individuals within our culturally heterogeneous society.

**SITUATION: The patient/family under care has significantly
different values and customs than the professional caregivers.**

Findings

- Initial and ongoing patient/family assessment reveal a wide range of cultural
differences, such as:
  - Country of origin, sense of nationality, ethnic background
  - Language, dress, interpersonal behavior, and interpretation of caregivers'
  spoken and "body" language (e.g., eye contact, "personal space," man-
  ners/mannerisms, etc.)
  - Attitudes toward individuality, autonomy, self-determination, and place
  within the family and society
  - Attitudes toward illness, dependency, dying, and death
  - Attitudes toward food, meals, and nutrition
  - Attitudes toward pain and suffering
  - Attitudes toward modesty and gender roles
  - Expression of spirituality: religion/religious institution, faith, rituals, beliefs

**Assessment, Processes of Care, Goals/Outcomes,
Documentation**

In order to provide meaningful end-of-life care, a thorough understanding of
the patient's/family's cultural imperatives and values is necessary. This may
be particularly challenging when there are language barriers, so every reasonable attempt should be made to obtain capable translation. If at all possible,
caregivers or volunteers should be assigned who have some experience with
the particular cultural values system of the patient/family, and the IDT can
then be better educated to the particular nuances that will affect care. Most
importantly, IDT members should ask patients and families *how they wish to be
cared for and if there is anything in their culture, religion, or tradition that the team
should be aware of in order to provide care desired by the patient and family.*

The entire hospice team needs to be committed to providing assistance
without prejudice to all people with limited life expectancy who want our help.
This mission demands the highest regard for individual rights and freedoms in
accordance with the laws of the land. Due to the diversity of people in our
society, it is more likely than not that we will encounter individuals who are very
different from ourselves. In order to be true to the principle of patient-centered
and family-focused care, insight into the values of those who invite us into this
phase of their lives is a necessity. Only through conscious attempts at understanding can unintended bias and unwitting "cultural blunders" be prevented.

It is beyond the scope of this manual to elaborate all the various cultural
differences that exist toward dying and death. Nevertheless, the hospice
professional is encouraged to expand his or her knowledge with an open-
minded and inquisitive attitude whenever the opportunity presents itself.
There are many resources for learning in every community: church groups,
cultural organizations, local libraries, and the Internet, among other sources,
can provide helpful background. And, under most circumstances, patients
and families are extremely pleased that someone is interested in seeing the
world through their eyes. Most important, your willingness to understand and

appreciate others' life views in the midst of their coming to terms with life and death will be valued beyond measure.

Denial

SITUATION: Problematic expressions of denial interfere with attainment of patient-directed goals, care of patient, ability to cope.

Findings

- Family insists that patient not be told prognosis.
- Resistance to accepting available support and help to the extent that inadequate care is rendered and patient goals cannot be realistically assessed/attained
- Preoccupation with somatic symptoms with a view toward re-diagnosis/cure in the face of appropriate diagnostic/prognostic information given
- Inability to acknowledge patient's physical and/or mental decline
- Excessive resistance to planning for future without patient, including final arrangements
- Excessive resistance to talk about prognosis
- Patient/family making unrealistic future plans
- Patient/family seems not to understand reason(s) for hospice referral, even though they have signed consent form.

Assessment

Psychosocial/Spiritual

- Explore and understand patient and caregiver's perception of situation.
- Explore and understand motivations for (purposes served by) denial.
- Assess history of coping style with prior losses.
- Assess impact of denial on family dynamics, symptom management, safety issues, and ability to cope.
- Review and understand cultural factors, beliefs/faith, and support systems of patient/caregiver/family.

Processes of Care

Practical

- Educate caregiver/family and care team about denial as a usual and healthy coping strategy, and the potential for maladaptive denial to interfere with good care and the attainment of goals.

Psychosocial/Spiritual

- Approach denial openly, thoroughly supporting it as a constructive self-protective coping mechanism.
- As appropriate, assist patient, caregiver, and family to confront the issues of denial and develop plans to achieve relief of unresolved concerns.

• Assist patient/caregiver to develop alternative constructive coping strategies as situation dictates.

Goals/Outcomes

• Patient/caregiver will address denial as barrier to patient care.
• Maladaptive coping styles will decrease, at least to the extent that adequate assessment of realistic and potentially attainable goals and care can take place.
• Patient/caregiver will more productively understand/utilize denial as an adjustment mechanism and as a response to loss to enhance remaining time before death.
• Patient/caregiver will make progress toward making final plans and funeral arrangements.

Documentation in the Medical Record

Initial Psychosocial/Spiritual Assessment

• Degree to which denial is playing a role in coping
• Evidence of maladaptive denial: interference with ability to adequately evaluate goals, expectations, hopes, etc.; interference with ability to ensure basic safety and/or quality care
• Risk for lack of closure and/or pathological grief

Interdisciplinary Progress Note

• Ongoing area(s) of denial
• Interventions and outcomes

IDT Care Plan

• Schedule of interventions: who, what, when
• Contingency plans if first set of approaches not beneficial
• Schedule of follow-up and reevaluation: who, when

Grief Reactions

SITUATION: Excessive grief interferes with patient's/caregiver's ability to function or cope.

Findings

• Excessive sadness, anger, guilt, anxiety, loneliness, fatigue, hopelessness, numbness (lack of attachment, dissociation), helplessness
• Sleep disturbance
• Eating disturbance
• Social withdrawal
• Restless or frenetic activity/compulsive or repetitive behaviors
• Somatic preoccupation, symptoms
• Mood disturbance (depression, mania)
• Impulsive behaviors

- Functional impairment
- Suicidal ideation
- Onset or exacerbation of addictive behaviors, including eating, smoking, alcohol abuse, gambling

Assessment

Biomedical

- Evaluate sleep patterns, eating patterns, mood, functional limitations, suicide risk.

Psychosocial/Spiritual

- Identify cultural background, traditions, and attitudes regarding death/grief.
- Understand spiritual beliefs/religious affiliation and practices.
- Understand how family expresses emotions and cultural norms for expressing grief.
- Define realistic parameters of life expectancy/prognosis.
- Determine the patient's role in the family and the potential impact of the loss.
- Review prior history of previous experiences with loss and coping style/ skills.
- Assess suicide potential/ideation.
- Assess support systems.
- Assess substance abuse, if indicated.

Interdisciplinary Team

- IDT to review, compare, and consolidate findings in order to determine the degree to which anticipatory grief is maladaptive and harmful

Processes of Care

Biomedical

- Treat disordered mood and sleep with appropriate medications on a short-term basis if not rapidly responsive to nonpharmacological approaches.
- Refer family member(s) to care of personal physician as appropriate.

Psychosocial/Spiritual

- Provide information on the grieving process.
- Encourage patient/caregiver to talk about his/her losses.
- Involve family in problem solving/goal setting.
- Assist patient/caregiver to identify and express emotions.
- Reinforce positive coping strategies.
- Suggest and help develop new or more adaptive coping strategies.
- Reinforce benefit of caregiver involvement in directly caring for patient and acknowledge/validate these efforts.
- Encourage participation in physical and social activities.
- Encourage expressive activities such as writing, painting, music, crafts, gardening, etc.
- Elicit preferences and facilitate family rituals.

Table 2.1 Grief and Bereavement in Children

Characteristics of Age	View of Death and Response	What Helps
BIRTH TO SIX MONTHS		
• Basic needs must be met, cries if needs are not met	• Has no concept of death	• Progressively disengage child from primary caregiver if possible.
• Needs emotional and physical closeness of a consistent caregiver	• Experiences death like any other separation—no sense of "finality"	• Introduce a new primary caregiver.
• Derives identity from caregiver	• Nonspecific expressions of distress (crying)	• Nurturing, comforting
• View of caregiver as source of comfort and all needs fulfillment	• Reacts to loss of caregiver	• Anticipate physical and emotional needs and provide them.
	• Reacts to caregiver's distress	• Maintain routines.
SIX MONTHS TO TWO YEARS		
• Begins to individuate	• May see death as reversible	• Needs continual support, comfort
• Remembers face of others, caregiver when absent	• Experiences bona fi de grief	• Avoid separation from close physical and emotional connections.
• Demonstrates full range of emotions, feelings, and interactions	• Grief response only to death of significant person in child's life	• Support caregiver to reduce distress and maintain a stable environment.
• Identifies caregiver as source of good	• Maintain daily structure and schedule	• Acknowledge sadness that loved one will not return—offer comfort.
• No control over feelings and responses; anticipateregressive behavior	• Screams, panics, withdraws, becomes disinterested in food, toys, activities	
	• Reacts in concert with distress experienced by caregiver	

TWO YEARS TO FIVE YEARS

• Egocentric	• Remind him or her that loved one will not return.
• Cause–effect not understood	• Give realistic information, answer questions.
• Developing conscience	• Involve in "farewell" ceremonies.
• Developing trust	• Help put words to feelings; provide ways to remember loved one.
• Attributes life to objects	• Keep home environment structured, stable.
• Feelings expressed mostly by behaviors	• Encourage questions, expression of feelings.
• Can recall events from past	• Reassure child who will take care of him or her.

FIVE TO NINE YEARS

• Attributes life to things that move; may fear the dark.	• Give clear and realistic information.
• Begins to develop intellect	• Include child in funeral ceremonies if he or she chooses.
• Begins to relate cause and effect; understands consequences	• Give permission to express feelings and provide opportunities; reduce guilt by providing factual information.
• Literal, concrete, may feel responsible	• Maintain structured schedule, individual and family activities.
• Decreasing fantasy life, increasing control of feelings	• Notify school of what is occurring, gentle confirmation, reassurance.
• Personifies death as ghosts, "bogeyman"	
• Interest in biological aspects of life and death	
• Begins to see death as irreversible	
• May see death as punishment; needs strong parent	
• Problems concentrating on tasks; may deny or hide feelings, vulnerability	

PREADOLESCENT THROUGH TEENS

• Individuation outside home	• Unambiguous information
• Identifies with peer group; needs family attachment	• Provide opportunities to express self, feelings; encourage outside relationships with mentors.
• Understands life processes; can verbalize feelings	• Provide tangible means to remember loved one; encourage self-expression, verbal and nonverbal.
• Physical maturation	• Dispel fears about physical concerns; educate about maturation; provide outlets for energy and strong feelings (recreation, sports, etc.); needs mentoring and direction.
• Views death as permanent	
• Sense of own mortality; sense of the future	
• Strong emotional reactions; may regress, revert to fantasy	
• May somaticize, intellectualize, morbid preoccupation	

- Mobilize bereavement support resources, including extended family, friends, community groups, religious organization or other spiritual care when valued by patient/caregiver/family.
- Facilitate funeral planning with patient/caregiver.
- Assist caregiver to explore ways to restructure life without patient.
- Identify complicated and pathological grief reactions and refer to appropriate mental health resource.
- Encourage participation in grief support programs.
- Consult with bereavement support staff.

Goals/Outcomes

- Patient/caregiver will verbalize understanding of normal grief response within cultural norms.
- Caregiver will utilize grief support services as appropriate.
- Patient/caregiver will express emotions related to grief.
- Patient/caregiver will verbalize sense of increased ability to cope with grief.
- Extreme and pathological grief reactions will be identified early so that appropriate resources can be mobilized.

Documentation in the Medical Record

Initial Psychosocial/Spiritual Assessment

- Grief reactions manifested by patient/caregiver

Interdisciplinary Progress Note

- Ongoing observations and evaluation of grief reactions
- Results of specific interventions

IDT Care Plan

- Specific interventions: who, what, when, how often
- Contingencies for poor response to primary interventions

NOTE: Processes of grief and bereavement in children depend on developmental age (Table 2.1). Anticipated and aberrant reactions must be readily distinguished and specially trained (pediatric) staff must intercede quickly when unhealthy behaviors are evident.

Living Environment, Finances, and Support Systems

SITUATION: Inadequacy of living environment, finances, or support systems interferes with patient care or ability of patient/caregiver to cope with illness/dying; self-neglect.

Findings

- No caregiver or frail or otherwise limited caregiver
- Insufficient food, heat, electrical power, protection from extremes of weather

- Infestation
- Poverty
- Hoarding
- Persistent inattention to personal hygiene and/or environment
- Repeated refusal of services that could reasonably be expected to improve quality of life
- Self-endangerment through the manifestation of unsafe behaviors
- Hazards (e.g., faulty wiring, heating, waste disposal/sanitation, or structures; unsecured weapons [guns, rifles, ammunition])
- Dangerous behaviors (e.g., smoking with oxygen or unattended while in bed)
- Isolation (e.g., inadequate transportation/telephone or inability to communicate due to language barrier or other communication problem)
- Insufficient financial resources for basic needs or expenses associated with illness and dying; inability to manage one's financial affairs
- Ongoing or imminent legal matters, disputes

Assessment

Psychosocial/Practical

- Assess ability of patient to have full capacity to live independently and assess insight into current situation and circumstances.
- Assess physical environment, and understand social support systems and extent of resources.
- Identify legal decision makers for patient.
- Understand needs and wants of patient/caregiver; desire to change.
- Define barriers to improving compromised situation.
- Define financial and practical needs: food, shelter, heating/cooling, phone, transportation, funeral and burial expenses, uncovered medical expenses, legal expenses.
- Determine unrealized sources of federal, state, and community assistance.
- Help to determine current and future expense, income, and assets.

Processes of Care

Psychosocial/Practical

- Address environmental concerns with patient/caregiver.
- Develop action plan among team to help make environmental improvements as acceptable to patient (utilize volunteers and community resource networks).
- Provide home safety education and plan.
- If safety and other basic concerns cannot be corrected, facilitate placement in a more secure environment if acceptable.
- Determine extent to which patient/caregiver will accept volunteers, home health aide, continuous care, and respite care to provide needed support.
- Provide information and help to procure financial assistance and social services, assist with application processes, and serve as liaison/facilitator/advocate with institutions and agencies.

• Explore guardianship, conservatorship, or special court proceedings if patient lacks capacity to manage affairs and/or medical care.

Recommended Reading

Reyes-Ortiz CA, Burnett J, Flores DV, Halphen JM, Bitondo Dyer C. Medical implications of elder abuse: self-neglect. *Clin Geriatr Med* 2014; 30(4):807–23.

Basic Home Safety

Environment

• Presence of weapons in the home
  • Ensure weapons are stored safely, secured in locked location, and stored separately from ammunition.
• Presence of pets in the home
  • Determine if there are health or safety risks and discuss with patient/caregiver and manage pets (especially dogs) to optimize well-being of patient and safety of professional caregivers (e.g., leashed, kenneled, etc.).
• Electrical safety: risk of electrical shock or fire
  • Remove electrical cords from beneath carpet and rugs.
  • Recommend replacement of worn, cracked, spliced, frayed electrical cords.
  • Reduce extension cord and multiple outlet adaptor overload.
• Floor safety: risk of falls and injury
  • Remove or secure loose rugs, runners, mats with appropriate fixation (tacks, adhesives, rubberized matting).
  • Secure loose carpet edges.
  • Recommend repair of uneven walkways or damaged flooring.
• Outside communication: help in case of emergency
  • If at all possible, place telephone where it is most accessible most of the time.
  • Emergency telephone numbers should be posted on or near telephone in large bold print.
• Fire safety
  • Recommend one smoke detector on every level of home.
  • Develop evacuation plan or review existing one with patient/caregiver; assign specific roles to capable live-in family members in case of fire.
  • Establish clear pathways to all exits.
  • Have key(s) accessible near key-locked (deadbolt) doors.
  • Inquire if actively used chimneys have been inspected; recommend annual inspection.
  • Kerosene heaters, woodstoves, and fireplaces should not be left unattended while in use.
• Bathroom safety
  • Tubs and showers should have nonskid surface/mats to prevent slips and falls.
  • Grab bars to assist transfers should be installed in tub, shower, and toilet area as needed.

- Adjust hot water heater temperature to avoid burns; check water temperature on sensitive body part before bathing/showering (patients with sensory neuropathy are particularly vulnerable).
- Use nightlights in the bathroom and hallways to bathroom.
- Bed safety
  - Assess need for pressure sore prevention and bed rails, and obtain safe/effective equipment as indicated.
- Stairs and passageway safety
  - Stairs, hallways, and passageways between rooms should be well lit and free of clutter.
  - Stairs should have sturdy, well-secured handrails on both sides.
  - Avoid using stairs while wearing only socks or smooth-soled shoes/slippers.
- Outdoors
  - Entrances should be clear of leaves, snow, and ice.
  - Recommend and assist with making arrangements to clear entryways in snowy weather.

Medical Supplies

General
- Storage
  - Keep supplies in a cool, dry, clean area protected from children and pets
- Handling
  - Make sure patient/caregiver has been given proper instruction on use and handling of all medical supplies and equipment, especially avoidance of injury and contamination
- Disposal
  - Instruct patient/caregiver that all dressing materials and disposable equipment that has been in patient contact should be wrapped in newspaper (if available), double bagged, and placed in a completely secure trash area

Oxygen
- Storage
  - Oxygen and tubing should be kept away from open flames or heat sources.
- Handling
  - Should be handled only by people who have been properly instructed by nursing personnel or medical equipment representatives
- Disposal
  - Used tubing should be disposed of in the manner described above.
  - All other equipment should be removed only by professional personnel.

Drugs
- Storage
  - Cool, dry place, secure from children and pets.
  - Determine the best balance between safety and convenience for the patient/caregiver.

- Determine whether medications require special handling or refrigeration. Review expiration dates.
- Handling
  - Ensure that all medications are adequately labeled.
  - **Check name, dose, and time schedule before giving/taking any medication.**
  - **Double check concentration of liquid medications and infusions; make sure that the dose per unit volume is exactly as intended; make sure the infusion rate is set to deliver the intended dose per unit time.**
  - Observe patient taking medications to determine independent capability.
  - Give instruction for refilling prescriptions on a schedule prior to using up current medication supply.
  - Count medication doses on a regular basis for those prescriptions to be taken on an "around the clock" schedule to ensure appropriate utilization.
- Disposal
  - Disposal methods for controlled substances: In September 2014, the Drug Enforcement Agency posted a final rule that reorganized and consolidated previously existing regulations regarding the disposal of controlled substances.
  - In the home setting, we are most concerned with "ultimate users," who are defined by the Controlled Substances Act (CSA) as a "person who has lawfully obtained, and who possesses, a controlled substance for his own use or for the use of a member of his household" (21 U.S.C. 802(27)). The rule provides three options for disposal by the ultimate user:
    1. Take-back events
    2. Mail-back programs
    3. Collection receptacles (The regulations provide specific language that continues to allow federal, state, tribal, and local law enforcement to maintain collection receptacles at law enforcement locations. Thus, family members should be able to contact their local law enforcement offices for locations and procedures.)
  - Hospice providers should be aware of these three methods of disposal and should be able to help family members choose the most appropriate method within the options available in a given community. In addition, hospice professionals should no longer recommend that controlled substances be flushed down the toilet. It is recommended that every hospice organization have a clear policy and procedure for controlled substance disposal consistent with these updated regulations, and that all staff are trained accordingly.
  - For a full description of disposal options in other settings (e.g., inpatient hospice units, long-term care facilities, and hospitals, please check the Federal Register: https://www.federalregister.gov/articles/2014/09/09/2014-20926/disposal-of-controlled-substances (last accessed April 19, 2016).
  - Remember, when in doubt, your contracted pharmacist is a wonderful source of information.

Needles and Syringes ("Sharps")

- Storage
  - Cool, dry place, secure from children and pets
- Handling
  - Examine for signs of contamination before opening.
  - All caregivers and patients need to be instructed in proper use, protection, and disposal.
  - Observe caregiver/patient capability prior to independent use.
- Disposal
  - Place used "sharps" in supplied puncture-resistant container to be returned to the hospice office for disposal.

Infectious Waste

- Storage
  - Do not store.
- Handling
  - Use gloves, confine to patient area, secure all materials in double plastic bags.
- Disposal
  - Flush all excretions/secretions down the toilet.
  - Dispose of contaminated materials as described above.
  - Cleanse reusable containers by soaking in a 1:10 dilution of household bleach for at least 30 minutes.

Parenteral and Enteral Solutions

- Storage
  - Store unopened enteral solutions/mixes at room temperature and administer at room temperature.
  - Opened cans or mixes for enteral feeding must be covered, dated and timed, and refrigerated and should be used within 24 hours of opening.
  - Parenteral solutions should be stored in a refrigerator (except lipids) and removed one hour prior to administration.
  - Parenteral solutions should be infused within 24 hours.
- Handling
  - Use clean technique when handling enteral solutions.
  - Use aseptic technique when handling parenteral solutions.
- Disposal
  - Dispose of all unused, partially used, or expired materials consistent with local ordinances and conventions. As environmental standards within communities become updated, an annual call to the state health department environmental office is recommended in order to maintain compliant policies and procedures.

Goals/Outcomes

- Develop a safe and comfortable environment for patient/caregiver and hospice staff.
- Appropriate use of medical equipment, supplies, and medications.

- Decrease financial and legal worries concerning patient care issues.
- Maintain patient/caregiver preferences and dignity as much as possible, balanced against safe working conditions for professional/volunteer staff.

Documentation in the Medical Record

Initial Psychosocial/Practical Assessment

- Determination of support systems
- Definition of financial and legal issues that may affect care
- Environmental assessment, risks, barriers to care

Interdisciplinary Progress Notes

- Instruction in basic safety measures (environmental, medical)
- Summation of discussions regarding options for environmental, financial, and legal help and patient/caregiver responses, preferences
- Description of interventions
- Results of interventions

IDT Care Plan

- Description of interventions: who, what, when
- Contingency and follow-up plans and alternatives based upon results of discussions/interventions and patient/caregiver response

Suicide: Risk Assessment, Prevention, and Coping If It Happens

SITUATION: Patient expresses thoughts or wishes for self-harm or suicide; or suicide occurs.

The risk of suicide is one of the most stressful and challenging situations clinicians face. The growing acceptance in the United States of physician-assisted death compounds the difficulty of addressing this issue. Nevertheless, cases of physician-assisted death are rare, and in the vast majority of states in the United States what people commonly think of as "suicide" (intentionally ending one's own life) is an occurrence that should be prevented, if at all possible. Assisting in another's life-ending action is illegal, except under the aegis of very specific and highly regulated statutory provisions.

Suicide is devastating to loved ones. It is irrevocable. And while no one can absolutely prevent another from taking her or his own life if he or she is determined to do so, what can be done in most instances are things that assist a suicidal person in reestablishing a more hopeful perspective with regard to his or her current circumstances.

Evidence suggests that most people who communicate the desire to end their life are highly ambivalent about going through with the act of killing themselves. It can be inferred that an inner voice is stating, "Please talk me out of this; please help me." With skillful, active, and empathic listening, coupled with other interventions, this help can be provided in most cases.

Findings

Warning Signs

Clinicians should look for warning signs of acute onset of suicidal behavior. The presence of any of these signs requires immediate attention. The observing clinician should immediately intervene by bringing in (other) members of the care team with expertise in this area. If need be, involvement with local emergency mental health services and/or inpatient care and monitoring should be sought.

- Threatening to hurt or kill self
- Looking for ways to kill self; seeking access to lethal means
- Talking or writing about suicide

Additional Warning Signs

- Assess for additional warning signs that can alert the clinician that a full assessment is indicated and that interventions need to be put in place to ensure safety:
  - Hopelessness
  - Feeling trapped—"no way out"
  - Withdrawing from family, friends, society
  - Anxiety, agitation, insomnia, hypersomnia
  - Dramatic changes in mood
  - Increasing alcohol or drug abuse
  - Rage, anger, seeking revenge
  - Acting recklessly, engaging in risky activities

Assessment

Assess for factors that may increase or decrease risk of suicide.

Biomedical

- Determine whether any physical symptoms are out of control.
- Assess patient/caregiver beliefs, perceptions about symptom-control issues.
- Assess impact of terminal diagnosis and fears related to disease progression.
- Review medications and determine if symptoms may reflect drug-related adverse effect.

Psychosocial/Spiritual

Factors That May Increase Risk

- Current ideation, intent, plan, access to means
- Previous suicide attempt(s)
- Previous history of psychiatric diagnosis, including alcohol/substance abuse
- Impulsiveness and poor self-control
- Hopelessness—presence, duration, severity
- Recent losses—physical, financial, personal
- Family history of suicide
- Recent discharge from a psychiatric inpatient unit

- History of abuse—physical, sexual, or emotional
- Comorbid health problems
- Age, gender, race—elderly or young adult, male, white, unmarried, living alone
- Same-sex sexual orientation

Factors That May Decrease Risk

- Positive social support
- Spirituality
- Sense of responsibility to family
- Children in the home
- Life satisfaction
- Reality testing ability
- Positive coping skills
- Positive problem-solving skills
- Positive therapeutic relationship

Specific Screening Questions

- Are you feeling hopeless about the present/future?
- Have you had thoughts about taking your life?
- When did you have these thoughts, and do you have a plan to take your life?
- Have you ever had a suicide attempt?

Full Assessment

A full assessment, completed by a trained social worker or other mental health professional, should include:

- Patient's current and past psychiatric diagnoses
- Patient/family history of suicide attempts and mental illness
- Individual strengths and vulnerabilities
- Acute and chronic stressors
- Current symptoms, complaints, and mental state

Processes of Care

Responding to Suicidal Risk

One of the most important steps that a clinician can take to address the potentially suicidal patient or family member is to establish a rapport with him/her that demonstrates trust and respect. There is no substitute for getting to know the person in crisis. This can be done even over the telephone on an initial contact by an on-call clinician if the proper skills, especially empathic listening, are utilized.

One way in which this can be done is by acknowledging the suffering that has led to thoughts of ending one's life. For a person in pain or anguish, knowing that someone is willing to "climb into the same hole" with them and attempt to see things from their perspective is comforting and an initial step toward building a relationship of trust and respect.

Once the foundations for this have been established, the clinician can proceed with the appropriate interventions based on assessed risk: to explore reasons to live and to develop a plan to address the concerns that have prompted the suicidal person to this point in his/her life.

NOTE: If, at any point during the assessment, the clinician determines that the risk of suicide is high, the clinician should consider immediate inpatient care or intervention of local emergency mental health resources. If risk is found to be moderate or low, the following interventions should be considered as part of the individual's treatment plan.

Biomedical

- Vigorously treat all out-of-control symptoms.
- Address high-risk symptoms of anxiety, agitation, and/or insomnia.
- Initiate antidepressant therapy if indicated and monitor closely (most will not have immediate effect; for patients with short life expectancy, consider psychostimulants).

Psychosocial/Spiritual

- Remove or secure lethal means of self-harm.
- Decrease isolation; involve family/friends; increase visit frequency of IDT.
- Add disciplines.
- Engage the individual in the development of a safety plan (see http://suicideline.org.au/at-risk/how-to-make-a-suicide-safety-plan).
  - Involve family/friends as appropriate.
  - Safety planning should include discussion and documentation of the following topics, and a copy should be given to the individual and/or family members as deemed appropriate:
    - Warning signs that a crisis may be developing
    - Coping strategies that the individual can use without needing to contact another person
    - Using contacts with people as a means of distraction from suicidal thoughts
    - Reasons for living; positive aspects of the individual's life
    - People the individual can contact who may help resolve the crisis
    - Professional contacts at hospice/palliative care or mental health agencies
    - How the individual's environment can be made safe; reducing potential for use of lethal means
- Refer for mental health assessment.
- Provide 24-hour contact (hospice number, suicide hotline, 911); consider continuous care if suicidal ideation increases.
- Focus on factors that are modifiable that can reduce risk of suicide.
- Enhance and provide support for protective factors that may reduce risk of suicide.
- Initiate psychotherapeutic interventions to manage high-risk factors of depression, hopelessness, and/or anxiety.
- Offer pastoral care or facilitate involvement with existing spiritual/religious leader; invite discussion about sense of meaning and purpose.
- Notify entire IDT and supervisor as to level of risk and need to monitor for increased risk.

- Explain limits of professional confidentiality applied to potential suicide.
- Instruct caregiver to observe for changes in mood or behavior and whom to notify.

Occurrence of Suicide

- Notify physician for appropriate completion of death certificate. Please note that although state laws can vary somewhat, deaths due to suicide typically require the involvement of the local medical examiner's office.
- Provide intensive bereavement support and counseling to family/caregiver.
- Refer family/caregiver to support groups as needed and per family preference.
- Provide "debriefing" and staff support for IDT members intimately involved in care.

Goals/Outcomes

- Identify factors that may increase or decrease an individual's level of suicide risk and estimate overall risk.
- Develop a plan of care that addresses safety and modifiable contributors to suicide risk.
- Enable patient's sense of purpose and meaning.
- Prevent suicide without stripping patient of dignity, autonomy, and rights of self-determination.
- Attain closure and functional grieving for family/caregiver and staff if suicide occurs.

Documentation in the Medical Record

Initial Biomedical Assessment

- Formal evaluation for symptom control and severe mood disorder

Initial Psychosocial/Spiritual Assessment

- Basis for determination of risk
- Changes made to plan of care and rationale for changes
- Safety plan
- Communication with and education of family members or caregivers

Interdisciplinary Team Notes

Results of discussions, reassessments, and specific interventions

IDT Care Plan

Specific interventions and contingency plans (who, what, when)
Follow-up plan

Recommended Reading

American Psychiatric Association. Practice guidelines for the assessment and treatment of patients with suicidal behaviors. In: *Practice Guidelines for the Treatment of Psychiatric Disorders Compendium*, 2nd ed., 2004:835–1027.

Department of Health and Human Services, Centers for Disease Control and Prevention, National Center for Health Statistics. *Medical Examiners' and Coroners' Handbook on Death Registration and Fetal Death Reporting*, 2003:21.

Department of Veterans Affairs Office of Inspector General. *Re-Evaluation of Suicide Prevention Safety Plan Practices in Veterans Health Administration Facilities*. 2004.Fochtmann LJ, Jacobs DG. Suicide risk assessment and management in practice: The quintessential clinical activity. *Acad Psychiatry* 2015; 39(4):490–491.

Haas A, Eliason M, Mays VM, et al. Suicide and suicide risk in lesbian, gay, bisexual, and transgender populations: Review and recommendations. *J Homosex* 2011; 58(1):10–51.

Section 3

Clinical Processes and Symptom Management

This section is organized alphabetically, for easiest access to subject matter. Although every effort has been made to ensure that *The Hospice Companion* is an evidence-driven clinical tool for use "at the bedside" and during care planning meetings, extensive referencing has been intentionally omitted. Instead, available literature has been synthesized and summarized in the form of treatment recommendations that are readily applicable in real-time instances. In lieu of a comprehensive bibliography, though, and both for integrity's sake and to satisfy the intellectual thirst of hospice professionals, every section ends with a recommended reading list consisting of seminal works and more contemporary literature that forms the basis of recommendations.

The *sine qua non* of quality hospice care in the 21st century is timely and effective pain and symptom management, conjoined with skilled expertise in emotional and spiritual counseling and support. Recognizing that people who are experiencing severe physical distress are unable to focus on other aspects of their existence, a major emphasis of this section is on interventions to reduce the physical burdens brought on by advanced illness. Ongoing refinements and specificity in pharmaceuticals and pharmacotherapy have served to enhance our abilities as hospice professionals to keep distressing symptoms associated with advanced disease under reasonable control in the vast majority of cases. Therefore, excellence in pharmacotherapy plays a critical role in the provision of high-quality hospice care, so solid grounding in this area is the starting point for the hospice clinician's knowledge base.

A fundamental principle of hospice is that all interventions, whether medication management or spiritual care, must be tailored to the individual needs and unique circumstances of each and every patient. With regard to pharmacotherapy (the medical keystone of pain and symptom management), the information provided in this section is meant to guide therapy and should not be used rigidly in lieu of clinical judgment. Pharmacoeconomics always plays a role in current-day health care, so cost considerations will enter into decision making at some level. These analyses should be used in order to make balanced decisions after sound assessment principles have been followed, leading to an indication for a therapeutic intervention.

Knowledgeable clinicians recognize that many symptoms (e.g., pain, anxiety, restlessness) have an often-lengthy differential diagnosis. For example, restlessness may reflect metabolic encephalopathy, air hunger (dyspnea), hypoxia, pain that is poorly localized or difficult to express, social stress, an unresolved emotional or spiritual issue, and so forth. Furthermore, each of these etiologies has its own lengthy differential diagnosis that may require further evaluation and specific treatment.

It is always incumbent on the clinician to make the best determination of the CAUSE of the distressing symptom in order to promote the best PALLIATION of the symptom. The more closely these are matched, the more likely it is that the patient's (and caregiver's) needs will be met. With this in mind, pharmacotherapy may not always be the best approach to symptom management. When it is, this guide should serve as a means of making this process more uniform and timely, actualizing the goals of maximizing therapeutic effect and minimizing adverse effects. Careful titration of drugs, especially when using polypharmacy (more than one drug at a time), is required to avoid toxic effects, especially when drug–drug interactions and synergistic effects are likely to occur. These should be understood, anticipated, prevented, and monitored. The effects of aging amplify many drug effects, and these principles and precautions should be accentuated in older individuals.

Because many symptom and treatment domains are overlapping (e.g., dysphagia and painful mucositis) cross-referencing will serve to make this resource as useful and compact as possible. When issues are not crystal clear, we can and should rely on the strength, diversity, and breadth of experience within the interdisciplinary team to find direction. True emergencies (e.g., pain out of control, extreme agitation, severe dyspnea) should trigger immediate intervention and, when necessary, consultation. For medically oriented problems, this guide should serve as a reference for immediate action, to relieve suffering as quickly as possible.

Clinicians should always choose the drug formulation that is believed to best serve the patient's needs, after all pertinent variables have been considered. Although clinical experience is invaluable, reliance on anecdotal experience alone is a dangerous trap. Generally speaking, extemporaneous formulations (compounding) should be avoided in favor of commercial formulations, because the latter are subject to considerable regulatory scrutiny and quality control, so factors such as dissolution and absorption are far more likely to be predictable. Last, expense is always a consideration in health care, and hospice in particular, due to its payment structure under the Medicare Hospice Benefit. Cost-effective therapies should drive clinical decision making, not cost containment. Good business practices combined with skilled case management should allow all patients to obtain the most beneficial treatments available in order to optimize therapeutic outcomes.

Agitation and Anxiety

SITUATION: Anxiety or agitation that is distressing to the patient/caregiver or negatively affects care of the patient or the caregiving environment.

Severe anxiety (or panic) and uncontrolled agitation represent some of the few, but true, emergency conditions (along with convulsions, hemorrhage, severe dyspnea, and pain) in the hospice setting. Anticipation and early recognition of these circumstances with a prevention and treatment plan are critical to optimal care of the dying.

Causes

Biomedical

- Respiratory distress (e.g., dyspnea from any cause; symptomatic hypoxemia and/or hypercarbia)
- Uncontrolled pain
- Primary anxiety/panic disorder
- Disease-induced psychosis (e.g., brain metastasis, metabolic disturbance)
- Drug-related psychosis (e.g., opioids, corticosteroids, medications with anticholinergic side effects)
- Sleep deprivation
- Agitated depression
- Full bladder, fecal impaction, nausea in a patient who cannot express distress other than through behavioral response
- Substance abuse/misuse/withdrawal (e.g., alcohol, opioid, benzodiazepine abstinence syndrome)

Psychosocial/Spiritual

- Response to imminent loss (anticipatory grief)
- Fear of the unknown and other fears associated with severe illness and imminent death
- Nightmares/night terrors

Findings

- Verbal or other expressions of anxiety, panic, terror, fear, worry
- Disordered sleep
- Misuse of prescribed medications and noncompliance with other treatment protocols
- Abusive language or behaviors toward caregivers
- Pressured speech, tangential thoughts, perseveration
- Volatile behavior; combative behavior
- Altered appetite
- Somatization
- "Panic" behaviors (e.g., frequent impulsive telephone calls, dialing 911)
- Increased complaints of pain despite appropriate analgesics
- Autonomic nervous system reactions (tachycardia, diaphoresis, tachypnea)
- Sense of impending doom or death without accompanying biomedical signs

NOTE: In advanced disease states, especially cancer, differentiating anxiety-related symptoms from somatic, visceral, or neurogenic manifestations of the disease may be extremely difficult. Empirical approaches to therapy may be required.

Assessment

The tactical approach to evaluating and managing severe anxiety and agitation should account for anticipated prognosis, the patient's treatment goals, and the caregiving environment.

Biomedical

- Evaluate for concomitant evidence suggesting an organic brain syndrome due to advancing disease with either local or systemic manifestations (e.g., hallucinations, nausea/vomiting, papilledema, hypo- or hyperglycemia, uremia).

NOTE: Laboratory testing should be done only if findings will specifically alter or influence the plan of care to alleviate distressing symptoms.

- Review medications for adverse drug reactions (e.g., psychotropic drugs, analgesics, corticosteroids, medications with anticholinergic side effects), with particular attention to following biochemical or physiological categories:
  - **Cholinergic deficiency** due to use of medications that are acetylcholine antagonists (anticholinergics): Examples include tricyclic antidepressants (e.g., amitriptyline), diphenhydramine; atropine and scopolamine; digoxin; furosemide.
  - **Dopaminergic excess**: medications used for Parkinson's disease or restless leg syndrome such as levodopa, pramipexole, ropinirole
  - **Neuroleptic malignant syndrome (NMS)**: This is an adverse reaction to antipsychotics. *NOTE: This is more likely to happen when there is rapid neuroleptic dose escalation and/or in patients dealing with Lewy Body dementia. This condition is associated with fever, autonomic instability, muscle rigidity, and delirium. Laboratory findings include elevated white blood cell count and creatine phosphokinase level due to rhabdomyolysis.*
  - **Serotonin syndrome**: This is due to serotonin toxicity as a result of overdose or drug–drug interaction(s) and can occur with any of the following medications: opioids, antidepressants, methylphenidate, triptans, lithium, dextromethorphan, antipsychotics, and certain antiemetics (e.g., ondansetron and metoclopramide). Like NMS, this syndrome manifests with autonomic instability and delirium. However, myoclonus and/or hyperreflexia are the third part of the symptom triad instead of fever or muscle rigidity.
  - **Akathisia**: This is a state of internal restlessness that can be triggered by antipsychotics, antidopamine antiemetics (e.g., metoclopramide and prochlorperazine), selective serotonin reuptake inhibitors (SSRIs) and other antidepressants, alcohol and drug withdrawal (particularly for opioids, benzodiazepines, and barbiturates), Parkinson's disease, and serotonin syndrome.
- Ensure that all medications whose abrupt discontinuation can lead to an acute abstinence syndrome are either maintained or slowly tapered (especially opioids, benzodiazepines, and psychoactive medications such as SSRIs).
- Inquire about ETOH history and last intake to assess for potential withdrawal.

- Inquire about and assess for infectious signs and symptoms, most notably referable to the urinary and respiratory tracts.
- Conduct systems review and examination of bladder and bowel function (e.g., urinary retention, constipation, fecal impaction).
- Examine less-than-fully coherent or noncommunicative patients for signs of unrecognized pain source (e.g., bone pain, abdominal pain, decubitus pain, etc.). This examination must include suprapubic palpation and a rectal examination—urinary retention and constipation are easily correctable causes of agitation in noncommunicative patients and must be recognized in a timely fashion!
- Respiratory examination for potential cause of hypoxemia/dyspnea (respiratory rate and pattern, use of accessory muscles, pallor/cyanosis, rales, pleural effusion)
- Cardiac examination for evidence of heart failure, ischemia, or arrhythmia (rate, rhythm, jugular venous distention, peripheral edema, rales, diaphoresis)

Psychosocial/Spiritual

- Patient self-rating on anxiety scale (if capable)
- Caregiver rating of patient on agitation scale
- Assess patient/caregiver perceptions of cause/source of anxiety/agitation.
- Review past experiences with significant losses and deaths.
- Review current and past history of anxiety/panic disorder and psychiatric care; refer to *Diagnostic and Statistical Manual, Fifth Edition (DSM-5)* for diagnostic criteria.
- Identify coping skills/social support and barriers to care.
- Observe interactions among caregiver(s) and patient.
- Assess impact of anxiety/agitation on overall care.
- Identify areas of unresolved conflict.

Processes of Care

Once the interdisciplinary team has identified the specific anxiety-related or agitation-related symptoms to be treated, a plan of care consistent with patient/family goals and values should be defined, explained, and implemented as quickly as possible.

Biomedical

- If hypoxemia-induced agitation responds to a trial of oxygen therapy, maintain oxygen administration protocol with usual recommendations and precautions.
- Attempt to reduce dyspnea by increasing air circulation with a portable fan.
- Listening-talking therapy should precede or supplement pharmacotherapy unless symptoms are immediately uncontrollable or at crisis levels.
- Nightmares or terrifying hallucinations and severe anxiety or agitation should be controlled emergently for the patient's and family's sake.
- In the noncommunicative patient with physical examination findings consistent with urinary retention, a Foley catheter may relieve the cause of agitation and obviate the need for pharmacological intervention.

- In the noncommunicative patient with physical examination findings consistent with constipation/fecal impaction, an aggressive bowel regimen (begin with a quick-acting intervention including manual disimpaction or an enema) may relieve the cause of agitation and obviate the need for further pharmacological intervention.

Pharmacotherapy for Acute and Recurrent Anxiety

1. Lorazepam 0.5 mg given by the oral (PO), sublingual (SL), subcutaneous (SQ), or intravenous (IV) route q2–4hr; titrate dose and interval as needed. Oral formulations of lorazepam (PO/SL) are considerably less costly than parenteral formulations. Sublingual lorazepam has been shown to be absorbed (attain plasma levels) similarly to parenteral administration.

2. In a crisis, without IV access, subcutaneous injection of lorazepam (1 to 2 mg) is the most expedient means to attain a calm setting in which to seek more specific treatment approaches (complete the assessment) or institute longer-term maintenance therapy.

3. Patients who are not responsive to low- or moderate-dose benzodiazepine therapy require further evaluation.

4. Patients who are responsive to low- or moderate-dose benzodiazepine therapy and who continue to have anxiety and have a prognosis of weeks to months may benefit from a daily antidepressant (SSRI [e.g., sertraline], serotonin–norepinephrine reuptake inhibitor [SNRI; e.g., venlafaxine], or buspirone).

Pharmacotherapy for Acute and Recurrent Agitation

NOTE: Before initiating pharmacotherapy, ensure that an easily correctable problem (e.g., urinary retention or constipation) is not the cause of agitation in a noncommunicative patient.

1. Mild or moderate restlessness or delirium: haloperidol 0.5 to 5 mg PO/SQ/IV q4–6hr (titrate upward as needed) or chlorpromazine 10 mg IV or 25 mg by the PO or rectal (PR) route q6–8hr (titrate upward as needed; SQ chlorpromazine should not be given because of skin irritation and risk of necrosis). In cases of Parkinson's disease the above antidopamine agents should be avoided due to the risk of exacerbating motor symptoms. Instead, titrate quetiapine 25 to 50 mg PO q6–12hr to efficacy.

2. More severe delirium and terminal restlessness (involuntary movements) often require more rapid dose titration and combination therapy. Paradoxical reactions to sedative drugs can occur; these effects should be recognized quickly so that alternative therapies can be instituted.

   a. Start with above-noted therapies (haloperidol or chlorpromazine plus lorazepam). If this is ineffective, consider adding phenobarbital 64.8 mg oral tab administered rectally or 65 mg IV/SQ administered q6hr as needed. Diphenhydramine 25 to 50 mg PO/IV q6hr should be used if extrapyramidal effects are noted when using haloperidol or chlorpromazine (avoid these antipsychotic drugs in patients with Parkinson's disease).

b. An expensive but effective alternative for control of terminal agitation symptoms that are poorly responsive to first-line therapies above is SQ/IV midazolam. It can be first given as a bolus dose of 2 to 5 mg followed by a continuous infusion of 1 mg/hr. Titrate up or down according to level of consciousness and emergence of symptoms. If a continuous infusion is not (immediately) possible, consider using an SQ port and administrating midazolam SQ q2–4hr scheduled or prn.

c. Another costly but effective treatment for total sedation in an inpatient setting is propofol infusion. This requires a central IV line and the supervision of a clinician experienced in using this medication to achieve and maintain sedation safely. Usual doses for initiating therapy are 10-mg (1-ml) incremental boluses in rapid succession (q1–5min, depending on patient's circulation time) until effective sedation is achieved without clinically significant respiratory depression. Continuous infusion at a rate of 10 to 50 μg/kg/hr is usually the effective range, but this must be titrated to individual circumstances and response. Propofol can be painful when infused through a peripheral vein. The addition of preservative-free lidocaine in a ratio of 40 mg lidocaine to 200 mg propofol (1 ml 4% lidocaine added to each 20 ml of propofol) is effective in eliminating pain during bolus or infusion.

Psychosocial/Spiritual

• Promote day and night routines that augment daytime activity and sleep.

• Minimize sensory impairment, immobility, or overstimulation when pertinent and fixable.

• Teach relaxation, imaging, and distraction techniques when applicable.

• Openly discuss feelings, perceptions, role changes, losses, and issues of control and frustration.

• Interact with patient/caregiver in a calm, reassuring manner.

• Use life review and storytelling techniques to engage patient and discern sources of conflict.

• Acknowledge and reduce fears and worries by providing information and clarifying distortions in thinking in a gentle and sensitive manner:
  • What can the patient/caregiver expect over the next days to weeks?
  • What is usual course of the disease and prognosis?

• Be open and invite all questions; look for the meaning behind "cloaked" questions.

• Reinforce coping skills and anxiety-reducing behaviors/techniques.

• Facilitate problem solving and decision making.

• Provide instruction on how to create a calm environment for patient and caregiver (be aware that paradoxical effects may occur—some people prefer chaos):
  • Reduce noise, bright light, clutter.
  • Increase structure, schedules, orderliness.
  • Limit physical restraints.

- Design crisis intervention plan for emergency management of out-of-control symptoms.
- Have pharmacotherapy orders available (see earlier under "Biomedical").
- Have hospice on-call telephone number immediately available.
- Hospice staff to consult with physician if symptoms do not respond to interventions within reasonable time period (1 to 4 hours, depending on severity of symptoms)

Goals/Outcomes

- Episodes of anxiety/agitation will be reduced in frequency and intensity in order to decrease distress to the patient and to alleviate caregiver burden.
- To establish clear communication with the family to ensure understanding of causes and treatments that are contextually appropriate and consistent with overarching goals and values
- To provide an opportunity for reconciling internal and interpersonal conflicts
- To eliminate the likelihood of self-harm or injury to caregivers
- To prevent avoidable transfers and discontinuity in care setting whenever possible

Documentation in the Medical Record

Initial Psychosocial/Spiritual Assessment

- Anxiety score recorded using standard analog scale (patient report)
- Agitation score recorded using standard analog scale (caregiver report)

NOTE: The CAM-S may be a useful way of capturing intensity of symptoms given patients' usual inability to report on such symptoms, with attention to acute onset or fluctuation, inattentiveness, disorganized thinking, and altered level of consciousness (see http://www.hospitalelderlifeprogram.org/delirium-instruments/ short-cam/short-cam-instrument/type/english/).

- Manifestations of anxiety/agitation
- Ability of caregiver to cope with patient's condition
- Social/environmental factors that contribute to anxiety/agitation

Initial Medical Assessment

- Medical findings and contributors to anxiety/agitation
- Physical manifestations of anxiety/agitation
- Effects of anxiety/agitation on medical condition
- Current medication and other substance use for pain, insomnia, restlessness, anxiety/agitation

Interdisciplinary Progress Notes

- Anxiety score recorded using 0-to-10 scale (patient report)
- Agitation score recorded using 0-to-10 scale (caregiver report)
- Patient/caregiver response to proposed interventions (e.g., agreement, denial, defensiveness, disregard, anger, etc.)
- Patient/caregiver compliance/acceptance of care plan
- Results of interventions and reassessments

- Proposed interventions: who, when, what
- Contingency plans and reassessment schedule
- Crisis prevention/intervention plan

Recommended Reading

Huh J, Goebert D, Takeshita J, et al. Treatment of generalized anxiety disorder: a comprehensive review of the literature for psychopharmacologic alternatives to newer antidepressants and benzodiazepines. *Prim Care Companion CNS Disord* 2011; 13(2): (nonpaginated).

Inouye SK, Kosar CM, Tommet D, et al. The CAM-S: Development and validation of a new scoring system for delirium severity in 2 cohorts. *Ann Intern Med* 2014; 160:526–533.

Lorenz RA, Jackson CW, Saitz M. Adjunctive use of atypical antipsychotics for treatment-resistant generalized anxiety disorder. *Pharmacotherapy* 2010; 30(9):942–951.

Maltoni M, Scarpi E, Rosati M, et al. Palliative sedation in end-of-life care and survival: a systematic review. *J Clin Oncol* 2012; 30(12):1378–1383.

Shub D, Ball V, Abbas AA, et al. The link between psychosis and aggression in persons with dementia: a systematic review. *Psychiatr Q* 2010; 81(2):97–110.

Air Hunger (Dyspnea)

SITUATION: Shortness of breath, chest tightness, and air hunger are often associated with findings of anxiety, panic, desperation, or impending doom.

This symptom is often more distressing than pain. Although it is very important to formulate a differential diagnosis as quickly as possible in order to match treatment with the identified cause whenever possible, **never delay palliative treatment for any reason.** Air hunger is probably the most terrifying symptom that can be experienced, and panic can overcome even the most stable and well-prepared patient, family, and other caregivers. THE EMERGENT TREATMENT OF CHOICE IS MORPHINE (OR ANOTHER RAPID-ONSET OPIOID IF THERE IS MORPHINE ALLERGY/SENSITIVITY), UNLESS A CAUSE IS IMMEDIATELY IDENTIFIED THAT CAN BE TREATED JUST AS QUICKLY. **ALTHOUGH BRONCHOSPASM, CONGESTIVE HEART FAILURE, AND OTHER CAUSES MAY ALSO REQUIRE EMERGENT TREATMENT, OPIOIDS SHOULD BE GIVEN CONCURRENTLY OR SHORTLY AFTER MEDICATIONS FOR THESE OTHER SPECIFIC CONDITIONS ARE GIVEN.** Fear of hypercapnia is often cited as a reason to delay use of opioids, but the literature consistently supports the safety of opioid use in dyspnea, when used at appropriate doses. The most rapid, readily accessible, and immediately available route of administration for morphine should be used.

For emergent/urgent treatment, choices include the following:

- Oral morphine concentrate (20 mg/ml): 1/4 to 1/2 ml (5 to 10 mg) SL/PO; repeat in 15 to 30 minutes as needed. May need higher doses in people with opioid tolerance, just as in pain management, and can use other opioids (for equianalgesic doses see "Pain" later in this section). Dose of opioids for prn use when tolerance is present is 10% to 15% of usual total 24-hour opioid dosage.

- Nebulized morphine (parenteral grade, preservative-free) 2.5 mg in 2 to 4 ml 0.9% (normal) saline or fentanyl 25 to 50 μg (1/2 to 1 ml) in the same volume of saline is an alternative if more readily available or if there is morphine sensitivity.

- Parenteral opioid delivery via the SQ route is feasible in most settings. For patients who have established IV access, it may be preferable and faster to titrate IV morphine, starting with 1 mg every few minutes in opioid-naïve patients, or an equivalent opioid (e.g., 10 μg fentanyl; 0.15 mg hydromorphone).

- The dose of opioid, regardless of route of administration, should be adjusted based on the previous experience and opioid tolerance of the patient.

- Benzodiazepines can also be used as adjuvants to opioids. Liquid lorazepam (2 mg/ml) can be given at a dose of 0.25 to 0.5 ml (0.5 to 1 mg) and repeated in 30 minutes as needed. Some studies have shown benzodiazepines to be equivalent or even superior to opioids in relieving dyspnea.

Causes

Practical

- Excessive or poorly regulated activity (pacing issues)
- Improper physical positioning (e.g., orthopnea)

Psychosocial/Spiritual

- Anxiety associated with dyspnea itself (i.e., a vicious cycle) or anxiety from other sources of worry, angst, etc., serving as a trigger for dyspnea
- Fear (usually compounded by experiences from previous episodes)
- Undertreated pain can cause anxiety, tachypnea, and dyspnea.

Biomedical

- Pulmonary disease (e.g., chronic obstructive pulmonary disease [COPD], restrictive lung disease, pneumonia)
- Pleural effusion
- Pericardial effusion
- Neuromuscular disease affecting coordinated mechanics of breathing and respiratory muscle function
- Uncompensated heart failure
- Weakness, fatigue, aesthenia due to primary disease or secondary causes (e.g., metabolic derangement, myasthenia)
- Anemia with inadequate oxygen-carrying capacity
- Acute pulmonary embolism (PE)
- Acute myocardial infarction (MI)

Findings

- Anxiety, restlessness, fearfulness, agitation, "panic facies"
- Complaint of shortness of breath or similar expression of breathing difficulties
- Inability to speak in complete sentences due to running out of breath
- Decreased functional ability due to shortness of breath
- Increased use of accessory muscles of respiration and posturing to catch breath (head forward, pursed-lip breathing, sitting bolt upright)
- Tachypnea
- Cyanosis, hypoxemia

Assessment

Practical

- Air circulation
- Dust, pollen, pet hair, strong perfumes/cleansers, etc.
- Patient positioning, availability of pillows, bolsters, etc.
- Assess bowel habits/constipation/stool impaction, especially if opioids are being used.
- Proximity of medications, caregiver
- Knowledge and understanding of crisis prevention plan

Biomedical

- Review diagnosis and likely medical etiologies for symptoms.
- Vital signs (respiratory rate, pattern, depth; pulse rate and quality; blood pressure [BP]; temperature)
- Cardiac examination: rate, rhythm, peripheral perfusion, venous distention
- Pulmonary examination: quality of breath sounds (wheezes, rales, rhonchi/rattles, acute changes)
- Extremity examination: edema, skin turgor, pallor
- Abdominal examination: acute distention, ascites, tenderness
- Check oxygen saturation (portable pulse oximeter) for acute changes.
- Patient self-rating of intensity/severity of episode(s) using a standardized numerical (0 to 10) scale (verbal or visual, depending on patient preference and capability) with 0 being "no shortness of breath" and 10 being "worst shortness of breath imaginable"; repeat measurements should be taken and noted after intervention(s); link patient/caregiver self-care and crisis prevention/intervention plan to severity ratings after some experience with this type of tool
- Occasionally, laboratory evaluation of hemoglobin/hematocrit to determine potential causes of limited oxygen-carrying capacity may be necessary if first-line palliative measures are not proving to be effective.

Psychosocial/Spiritual

- Acquire history of previous experiences, interventions, worries, plan for preventing crises, and potential emotional triggering factors.

Processes of Care

Practical

- Avoid gas-forming foods to prevent gastric/bowel distention.
- Discuss and facilitate remedial environmental adjustments to decrease symptom triggers and improve respiratory mechanics (e.g., rest periods, pacing, raise head of bed, use of bolsters, etc.).
- Instruct patient/caregiver in optimal patient positioning, day and night.
- Provide durable medical equipment (DME) as needed for positioning.
- Provide air movement using a fan and/or humidifier if at all possible, and determine symptomatic utility.
- Teach percussion and vibration to caregiver(s) as indicated.
- Devise crisis prevention and care plan.
- Review regularly what to do and when and whom to call.
- Check patient/caregiver understanding.
- Optimize accessibility and availability of prophylactic/therapeutic/communication resources.

Biomedical

- Notify physician of any unexpected or significant changes in physical examination that may require change in care plan or physician evaluation.
- Institute oxygen therapy ONLY if demonstrated that patient is hypoxemic AND there is a therapeutic response to the use of supplemental oxygen. Otherwise, use personal fans or other means of increasing air circulation.
- Optimize medical management (diuretics, vasodilators, bronchodilators).
- Consider trial of passive positive pressure (external) breathing device, if available.
- Palliative pharmacotherapy
  - Primarily anxiety-triggered dyspnea
    — Anxiolytic therapy: lorazepam PO/SL/SQ 0.5 to 2 mg q2–4hr or prn is given
    — NOTE: Titrate dose slowly to effect, especially when using in combination with opioids, to determine patient's sensitivity.
  - Primarily non–anxiety-triggered dyspnea
    — Opioid therapy: Rapidity of onset and therapeutic effect is a function of establishing blood levels as quickly as possible.
      • For patients with IV access, titrate IV doses to effect q15 min (e.g., morphine sulfate 1 mg or equivalent) to determine patient's sensitivity and threshold for response.
      • For patients without IV access, similar SQ doses can be given, or administer oral morphine concentrate (20 mg/ml) titrated to effect, starting with 0.25 to 0.5 ml SL/PO. Alternatively, nebulized morphine 2.5 mg in 2 to 4 ml 0.9% (normal) saline or fentanyl 25 to 50 μg in the same volume of saline is recommended. The medical literature is inconclusive about this form of therapy, but anecdotal experience has been favorable in some patients, especially as an alternative

to establishing IV access or much slower absorption routes (SQ/SL). This symptom should be anticipated in susceptible patients so that the apparatus for nebulizer treatments is readily available.
- An alternative to nebulized or parenteral drug delivery in order to establish rapid patient-controlled levels of opioid is fentanyl via the buccal or SL route. Various formulations are available, as either a lozenge on a stick, dissolvable tablets (buccal and sublingual), buccal patches, or sublingual and nasal sprays. It is recommended to start at the lowest available dose (100 or 200 µg) ONLY IN OPIOID-TOLERANT PATIENTS; this provides opioid-tolerant patients a noninvasive, self-administered means of relieving dyspnea for those without IV access, SQ dosing, or immediate access to nebulizer set-up. There is limited clinical experience with this technique.
— Recurrent episodic therapy with opioid analgesics by the most convenient route with an anxiolytic (lorazepam PO/SL/SQ 0.5 to 2 mg q2–4hr or prn) is usually necessary until death unless there is a well-defined remediable cause (see below).

Treatable Causes
1. Bronchospasm: A history of asthma or COPD is usually present. Listen for expiratory wheezes. Use a nebulized β_2-agonist (e.g., albuterol). Inhaled corticosteroids (e.g., beclomethasone) are proving to be beneficial in relieving acute bronchospasm. Systemic corticosteroids (e.g., prednisone) may be required in refractory cases.
2. Pulmonary edema due to congestive heart failure (CHF): Volume overload and left ventricular failure, leading to right ventricular failure, are the most common causes. Restriction of fluids and limiting sodium intake (or artificial feedings) and use of morphine therapy may relieve acute symptoms. In refractory cases, consider initiating or advancing diuretic therapy (furosemide 40 to 240 mg), inotropic therapy (digoxin), and angiotensin-converting enzyme (ACE) inhibitor therapy, according to clinical signs and symptoms, assessed by auscultation of heart and lungs, jugular venous distention, peripheral edema, and balance of fluid intake and (urinary) output.
   - In severe cases, where urgent palliation is indicated, parenteral diuretic and opioid drug administration is warranted, by the most convenient route (IV, intramuscular [IM]). For truly intractable cases of dyspnea due to CHF, IV milrinone (although very expensive compared to opioids and benzodiazepines) has been found to be effective.
3. Bronchial obstruction by tumor: Consider radiation therapy if prognosis allows; corticosteroid therapy for end-stage palliation (e.g., dexamethasone up to 12 mg/day in divided doses); and for symptomatic relief, nebulized fentanyl and lidocaine have also been used with varying degrees of efficacy.
4. Pleural effusion: Consider thoracentesis only if symptoms are not readily managed by noninvasive means (opioid and benzodiazepine pharmacotherapy, positioning, diuretics) and there is likelihood of significant improvement in performance status or return to a level of functioning meaningful to the patient. In the final days of life, thoracentesis

(especially if not able to be performed in the home) adds a greater burden than benefit. If nonloculated peripheral pleural effusions recur within days, and the relief of symptoms was viewed as meaningful to the patient, consideration for pleurodesis is appropriate in patients with a life expectancy of more than a few weeks.

5. Superior vena cava syndrome (obstruction of the superior vena cava): dexamethasone 24 mg IV followed by aggressive symptom control with corticosteroid, opioid, and benzodiazepine pharmacotherapy while considering the merits of radiation therapy (for patients with an otherwise predicted life expectancy of more than a few weeks)

6. Ascites: Diuretic therapy (e.g., furosemide 40 mg PO and spironolactone 100 mg PO per day, titrated upward as needed to maximum daily doses of furosemide 240 mg, spironolactone 400 mg) is the first line of therapy. However, diuretics are rarely helpful in cases of malignant ascites. In terminal disease states, paracentesis is rarely indicated. In cases of slowly developing ascites leading to dyspnea, where the burdens of symptom-relieving pharmacotherapy (opioids plus benzodiazepines) seem to outweigh the benefits, paracentesis should be considered if there is a life expectancy of several days to weeks.

7. Secretory conditions: Consider scopolamine SQ (0.2 to 0.4 mg) or transdermal; or glycopyrrolate 0.2 mg SQ and saline nebulizer treatments.

Psychosocial

- Teach relaxation techniques, cognitive-behavioral techniques, and breathing exercises.
- Address worries and fears in a direct, supportive way; help solve problems when concrete issues arise.
- Reduce anxiety by assuring patient and caregiver that measures to improve symptoms will be taken immediately.

Goals/Outcomes

- Reduced frequency and intensity of dyspneic episodes, with concurrent decrease in distress
- Improved sleep, appetite (if applicable), social interaction, mood, interest in what life has to offer
- Improved functional status (if applicable) (e.g., self-care, time out of bed, toileting out of bed, etc.)
- Decreased work of breathing
- Elimination of crises and unwanted interventions and transfers (e.g., ambulance calls, emergency department visits, hospitalizations, intubation, etc.)

Documentation in the Medical Record

Initial Medical Assessment

- Pertinent systemic review, examination findings, diagnostic impressions
- Dyspnea rating (patient self-report)

Initial Practical/Psychosocial/Spiritual Assessment

- Nonmedical initiating and contributing factors

Interdisciplinary Progress Notes

- Results of interventions
- Changes in biomedical, psychosocial, spiritual issues and circumstances influencing symptoms and management
- Repeat dyspnea ratings (patient self-report)

IDT Care Plan

- Nonpharmacological and pharmacological interventions with appropriate medical orders
- Follow-up and contingency plans
- Crisis prevention/intervention plan

Recommended Reading

Abernethy AP, McDonald CF, Frith PA, et al. Effect of palliative oxygen versus room air in relief of breathlessness in patients with refractory dyspnoea: a double-blind, randomised controlled trial. *Lancet* 2010; 376(9743):784–793.

Cranston JM, Crockett A, Currow D. Oxygen therapy for dyspnoea in adults. *Cochrane Database Syst Rev* 2008 Jul 16;(3):CD004769.

Currow DC, Agar M, Smith J, Abernethy AP. Does palliative home oxygen improve dyspnoea? A consecutive cohort study. *Palliat Med* 2009; 23(4):309–316.

Currow DC, Smith J, Davidson PM, et al. Do the trajectories of dyspnea differ in prevalence and intensity by diagnosis at the end of life? A consecutive cohort study. *J Pain Symptom Manage* 2010; 39(4):680–690.

Freeman S, Hirdes JP, Stolee P, et al. Correlates and predictors of changes in dyspnea symptoms over time among community-dwelling palliative home care clients. *J Pain Symptom Manage* 2015; 50(6):793–805.

LeBlanc TW, Abernethy AP. Building the palliative care evidence base: lessons from a randomized controlled trial of oxygen vs room air for refractory dyspnea. *J Natl Compr Canc Netw* 2014; 12(7):989–992.

Mahler DA, Selecky PA, Harrod CG, et al. American College of Chest Physicians consensus statement on the management of dyspnea in patients with advanced lung or heart disease. *Chest* 2010; 137(3):674–691.

Navigante AH, Castro MA, Cerchietti LC. Morphine versus midazolam as upfront therapy to control dyspnea perception in cancer patients while its underlying cause is sought or treated. *J Pain Symptom Manage* 2010; 39(5):820–30.

Silvestre J, Montoya M, Bruera E, Elsayem A. Intensive symptom control of opioid-refractory dyspnea in congestive heart failure: Role of milrinone in the palliative care unit. *Palliat Support Care* 2015; 13(6):1781–1785.

Anorexia and Cachexia

SITUATION: Progressive decline in appetite, nutritional status, and body mass as a result of catabolic changes associated with chronic disease.

Approximately 80% of people with advanced disease suffer from these debilitating and often demoralizing consequences of cancer and other chronic disease states. Despite the high prevalence of hospice patients who are affected by anorexia and cachexia, uniform definitions of these often-coexisting conditions have not been agreed upon. Clinically useful definitions for the hospice clinician include the following:

- Anorexia is the uncontrolled lack or loss of appetite for food.
- Cachexia is involuntary weight loss.
  - Specifically, it is defined as the loss of muscle with or without loss of fat mass.
  - Cancer anorexia–cachexia syndrome (CACS) is the loss of muscle mass (with or without loss of fat mass) that leads to progressive functional impairment despite optimal nutritional support. It is defined by involuntary weight loss of more than 5%, or more than 2% if the patient suffers from low body mass index (BMI < 20 kg/m^2) or decreased skeletal muscle mass (sarcopenia).
  - The cause is complex and characterized by hypercatabolism and systemic inflammation. In addition, patients suffer from reduced nutritional intake and increased resting energy expenditure.

Causes

Biomedical

- Cancer: especially common in tumors of the head and neck, gastrointestinal (GI) tract, pancreas, central nervous system (CNS), and lungs
- Cardiac disease
- Chronic kidney disease
- COPD
- HIV/AIDS
- Rheumatoid arthritis

Findings

- Decreased or no appetite with lack of interest in eating
- Feeling of fullness after ingestion of minimal food (early satiety) that may result from organomegaly ("squashed stomach")
- Persistent nausea
- Lack of taste perception (ageusia) and distortion of taste perception (dysgeusia)
- Dehydration, uremia, hypercalcemia, and other metabolic alterations
- Oral candidiasis, mucositis, and cheilitis (redness/swelling of the lips)
- Gastritis

Assessment

Practical

- Environmental assessment to determine source(s) of unpleasant odors
- Determine food preferences, reactions to various foods (what is particularly pleasant/unpleasant), and recent food intake, as well as past and present patterns of hunger/eating.
- Identify practical and functional limitations such as ability to chew and swallow, use of dentures, etc.
- Determine patient/caregiver understanding and capability to prepare modified foods (e.g., blended, pureed), if there are barriers to obtaining

foods (e.g., transportation, finances), and any practical limitations of food storage or preparation (e.g., refrigeration, cooking, infestation).

Biomedical

- Identify underlying causes or contributing factors that may be subject to palliation, correction, or treatment if the patient's sense of well-being is negatively affected by signs/symptoms:
  - Pain
  - Nausea
  - Uremia, hypercalcemia, hypogonadism, and thyroid dysfunction
  - Constipation, obstipation, impaction
  - Bowel obstruction
  - Hepatomegaly
  - Depression
  - Oral candidiasis
  - Mucositis, esophagitis, gastritis
  - Xerostomia (dry mouth)
- Assess patient's ability to swallow.
- Computed tomography (CT), magnetic resonance imaging (MRI), and dual-energy X-ray absorptiometry (DXA) are accurate ways of determining body composition and identifying muscle wasting (sarcopenia). However, cost limits their applicability in the clinical setting.
  - Multiple studies have shown a link between sarcopenia and functional status, chemotherapy toxicity, time to tumor progression, and mortality.

Psychosocial/Spiritual

- Assess symbolic value of nutrition/hydration to patient/caregiver (nurturing, guilt) and identify areas of patient/caregiver conflicting opinions, beliefs, or values related to feeding/hydration.
- Determine to what degree anorexia/cachexia signs and symptoms are disturbing to patient/caregiver and what preferences/goals/concerns exist about these.

Processes of Care

Practical

- Reduce environmental factors that negatively influence patient's interest/enjoyment in meals, and suggest enhancements such as the following:
  - Make an effort to take meals in esthetically pleasing environment with companionship rather than in bed or sleeping area.
  - Have patient suck on hard candy (trial and error of sweet vs. sour/citrus) to mask bad tastes.
  - Involve patient in menu planning.
  - Try very small portions with more frequent feedings, if patient is interested.
  - Suggest cold (semifrozen) nutritional drinks to overcome difficulties with chewing, swallowing, and odor/taste aberrations if patient is interested.
  - If acceptable and tolerated, consider a preprandial alcoholic beverage of choice (alcohol is an appetite stimulant).

Biomedical

- Inform patient/caregiver of relative risks/burdens versus benefits of various routes of alimentation and hydration as applicable.
- Palliative pharmacotherapy
  1. Corticosteroids: Multiple studies have shown a benefit in appetite stimulation. Side effects with long-term use include immunosuppression, myopathy, insulin resistance, Cushingoid facies, and adrenal insufficiency. There is no consensus on dosing, but suggestions are as follows:
     a. Dexamethasone 4 to 8 mg PO q day. Consider single a.m. dose to decrease risk of insomnia.
     b. Methylprednisolone 8 to 16 mg PO bid
     c. Prednisone 5 mg PO tid
  2. Hormonal therapy: Megestrol acetate is the only noncorticosteroid hormonal therapy showing a positive appetite stimulation effect, accompanied by a slight weight gain. However, increased mortality, edema, and thromboembolism were also seen. Risks and benefits of treatment should be discussed with patients prior to initiating therapy.
     a. Megestrol acetate 80 to 160 mg PO qid (study doses ranged from 400 to 800 mg PO per day in divided doses)
  3. Other approaches
     a. Dronabinol 2.5 mg PO bid or tid; has not been shown to be effective in CACS patients with advanced cancer but is effective in advanced HIV disease
     b. Cyproheptadine 8 mg PO tid; mild stimulatory effect on appetite in CACS patients, but no effect on weight loss
     c. Thalidomide has been found to reduce anorexia/cachexia associated with HIV disease. Evidence for benefit in cancer patients is conflicting. Use is limited by high cost.
  4. Investigative therapies
     a. Ghrelin and ghrelin receptor agonists (e.g., anamorelin) stimulate secretion of growth hormone and cause increased food intake and weight gain. Small, preliminary studies have shown increased body weight and increased appetite.
     b. Eicosapentaenoic acid (EPA) is an alpha-3 omega fatty acid found in fish oil. Data are conflicting on its beneficial effects. More research is needed.
     c. Immunomodulators (e.g., etanercept and infliximab) target the inflammatory process of anorexia–cachexia. Small studies have failed to show effectiveness. Many new research studies are focusing on combination therapy to target multiple pathways of inflammation.
     d. In theory, physical exercise may slow progression of cachexia by decreasing muscle loss, increasing insulin sensitivity, and lowering systemic inflammation. However, randomized controlled trials need to be done to determine its effectiveness.

Psychosocial/Spiritual

- Reassure patient/caregiver/family that anorexia/cachexia are usual occurrences associated with progressive chronic diseases.

- Help open up discussion regarding any conflicts that may exist concerning nutrition and hydration.
- Educate and dispel myths about utility of alimentation (enteral or parenteral) under conditions of "wasting" diseases.
- Discuss ethical/moral concerns regarding alimentation and hydration in the face of life-limiting illness.

Goals/Outcomes

- Amount, frequency, and type of alimentation/hydration will be commensurate with attainable preferences/goals of patient and appropriate to disease state.
- Decrease symptoms attributed to or associated with anorexia/cachexia that are disturbing to patient.

Documentation in the Medical Record

Initial Practical/Psychosocial/Spiritual Assessment

- Findings related to environmental factors contributing to troublesome symptoms
- Elaboration of issues pertaining to preferences, goals, and values related to alimentation/hydration; copy and place specific advance directives in chart

Initial Medical Assessment

- Review of systems and history pertaining to and associated with anorexia/cachexia
- Physical findings, stage of disease, nutritional status
- If available, imaging studies may yield helpful information.

Interdisciplinary Progress Notes

- Description of interventions
- Results of interventions
- Ongoing evaluation of mental and physical status

IDT Care Plan

- Timing of interventions, visits, and contingency plans
- Medical orders for pharmacotherapy

Recommended Reading

Chasen M, Hirschman SZ, Bhargava R. Phase II study of the novel peptide-nucleic acid OHR118 in the management of cancer-related anorexia/cachexia. *J Am Med Dir Assoc* 2011; 12(1):62–67.

Fearon K, Strasser F, Anker SD, et al. Definition and classification of cancer cachexia: an international consensus. *Lancet Oncol* 2011; 12(5):489–495.

Gabison R, Gibbs M, Uziely B, Ganz FD. The Cachexia Assessment Scale: development and psychometric properties. *Oncol Nurs Forum* 2010; 37(5):635–640.

Garcia JM, Boccia RV, Graham CD, et al. Anamorelin for patients with cancer cachexia: an integrated analysis of two phase 2, randomised, placebo-controlled, double-blind trials. *Lancet Oncol* 2015; 16(1):108–116.

Granda-Cameron C, DeMille D, Lynch MP, et al. An interdisciplinary approach to manage cancer cachexia. *Clin J Oncol Nurs* 2010; 14(1):72–80.

Grande AJ, Silva V, Riera R, et al. Exercise for cancer cachexia in adults. *Cochrane Database Syst Rev* 2014;(11): CD010804.

Holmes S. A difficult clinical problem: diagnosis, impact and clinical management of cachexia in palliative care. *Int J Palliat Nurs* 2009; 15(7):322–326.

Hopkinson JB, Fenlon DR, Okamoto I, et al. The deliverability, acceptability, and perceived effect of the Macmillan approach to weight loss and eating difficulties: a phase II, cluster-randomized, exploratory trial of a psychosocial intervention for weight- and eating-related distress in people with advanced cancer. *J Pain Symptom Manage* 2010; 40(5):684–695.

Kwang AY, Kandiah M. Objective and subjective nutritional assessment of patients with cancer in palliative care. *Am J Hosp Palliat Care* 2010; 27(2):117–126.

Miller S, McNutt L, McCann MA, McCorry N. Use of corticosteroids for anorexia in palliative medicine: A systematic review. *J Palliat Med* 2014; 17(4):482–485.

Prado CM, Birdsell LA, Baracos VE. The emerging role of computerized tomography in assessing cancer cachexia. *Curr Opin Support Palliat Care* 2009; 3(4):269–275.

Reid J, Mills M, Cantwell M, et al. Thalidomide for managing cancer cachexia. *Cochrane Database Syst Rev* 2012;(4): CD008664.

Ruiz Garcia V, López-Briz E, Carbonell Sanchis R, et al. Megestrol acetate for treatment of anorexia-cachexia syndrome. *Cochrane Database Syst Rev* 2013;(3): CD004310.

Belching and Burping (Eructation)

SITUATION: Distress, discomfort, or abdominal pain associated with frequent belching, burping, distention, or bloating.

Causes

Biomedical

- Aerophagia (air swallowing; may be secondary to anxiety with associated accumulation of esophageal and gastric gas)
- Supragastric belching (swallowing air into esophagus and immediately belching, often repetitive)
- Dysfunctional swallowing (cranial nerve or motor impairment)
- Gastric reflux/indigestion
- Gastroparesis, ileus, or small bowel obstruction
- Excessive oral secretions or difficulty managing secretions

Psychosocial

- Anxiety

Findings

Biomedical

- Feeling of epigastric or substernal fullness/pressure; excessive pressure may refer pain to chest or cause esophageal reflux with symptoms of "heartburn"

- Nausea/vomiting/regurgitation/odor
- Abdominal distention (tympany; diminished or excessive bowel sounds [borborygmi])
- Oral lesions and/or excessive secretions
- Impaired swallowing/choking

Psychosocial

- Anxiety related to pain, pressure, bloating
- Embarrassment around altered body function, odor
- Social isolation due to impaired eating and embarrassment

Assessment

Biomedical

- Review nutritional status and food intake as cause of excessive gas production (carbonated beverages, dairy products, fats, mints, chocolate).
- Assess and rule out bowel dysmotility, masses.
- Examine oropharynx, cranial nerves, and swallowing action.

Psychosocial

- Patient self-rating on anxiety scale (if capable)
- Caregiver rating of patient on agitation scale
- Determine the degree of distress symptoms are causing patient and family; this will help determine how aggressively symptom management should be approached.
- Assess patient/caregiver perceptions of cause/source of anxiety/agitation if these emotional factors are believed to be contributory or perpetuating.
- Identify coping skills, social support, and barriers to care.
- Observe interactions among caregiver(s) and patient.
- Assess impact of symptoms on overall ability to meet other care goals.

Processes of Care

Biomedical

- For isolated excessive belching due to air swallowing, behavioral therapy has been shown to decrease symptoms.
- Consider Speech Therapy to evaluate and educate patient and family.
- Evidence of bowel obstruction or ileus should be immediately brought to the attention of the physician before instituting any other therapy.
- Patient education about avoiding air swallowing and avoiding carbonated beverages
- Adjust positioning in bed to elevate head to at least 30 degrees to promote gastric gas to move into the small intestine.
- Dietary instruction to avoid foods that cause indigestion or are difficult to chew and swallow; encourage smaller, more frequent meals
- Avoid foods with prolonged transit times such as fats.
- Instruct patient to thoroughly chew simethicone tablets, if able.
- Pharmacotherapy

1. Simethicone 80-mg chewable tablets: Instruct patient to chew 2 to 4 tablets thoroughly as needed after meals and at bedtime, not to exceed 6 tablets per day.
2. Consider trial of H2 blocker or proton pump inhibitor (PPI) on a limited basis.
3. For anxiety-related symptoms, refer to "Agitation and Anxiety" earlier in this section.
4. For related oropharyngeal problems, refer to "Dysphagia and Oropharyngeal Problems" later in this section.

Psychosocial

- Teach relaxation, imaging, and distraction techniques when applicable.
- Reinforce coping skills and anxiety-reducing behaviors/techniques.

Goals/Outcomes

- Relieve distention and excessive belching
- Reduce physical and psychological distress

Documentation in the Medical Record

Initial Medical and Psychosocial Assessment

- Potential cause(s) of eructation
- Physical examination findings (cranial nerves, swallowing, oropharynx, larynx, trachea, and abdomen)
- Amount of distress/discomfort caused by symptoms
- Remedies tried by patient/caregiver with degree of success

Interdisciplinary Progress Notes

- Results of selected interventions and ongoing assessments

IDT Care Plan

- Interventions and contingency plans

Recommended Reading

Bredenoord AJ, Smout AJ. Physiologic and pathologic belching. *Clin Gastroenterol Hepatol* 2007; 5(7):772–775.

Bredenoord AJ, Weusten BL, Sifrim D, et al. Aerophagia, gastric, and supragastric belching: a study using intraluminal electrical impedance monitoring. *Gut* 2004; 53(11):1561.

Hemmink GJ, Bredenoord AJ, Weusten BL, et al. Supragastric belching in patients with reflux symptoms. *Am J Gastroenterol* 2009; 104(8):1992–1997.Hemmink GJ, Ten Cate L, Bredenoord AJ, et al. Speech therapy in patients with excessive supragastric belching—a pilot study. *Neurogastroenterol Motility* 2010; 22(1):24–28.Kessing BF, Bredenoord AJ, Smout AJ. The pathophysiology, diagnosis and treatment of excessive belching symptoms. *Am J Gastroenterol* 2014; 109(8):1196–1203.

Koukias N, Woodland P, Yazaki E, Sifrim D. Supragastric belching: prevalence and association with gastroesophageal reflux disease and esophageal hypomotility. *J Neurogastroenterol Motility* 2015; 21(3):398–403.

Montalto M, Di Stefano M, Gasbarrini A, Corazza GR. Intestinal gas metabolism. *Digest Liver Dis* 2009; 3(2):27–29.

Bleeding, Draining, and Malodorous Lesions

SITUATIONS:

- Minor, moderate, or major bleeding leading to patient and caregiver distress, fatigue (anemia), and excessive caregiver burden
- Malodorous and draining lesions causing significant social, emotional, and physical distress for patients and caregivers. Such lesions are a constant reminder of disease progression. The overwhelming smell can cause even the most loving of family members and caregivers to avoid contact with the patient. A malodorous draining wound may completely alter a patient's self-image, causing him/her to feel embarrassed, isolated, and unlovable. Of all of the symptoms associated with malignant wounds, malodor causes the most distress to patients, caregivers, and families. That is why it is so vital to do everything possible to alleviate this most burdensome of situations.

Causes

- Nonhealing wounds: breakdown of skin integrity, poor nutritional status, improper positioning, inadequate blood supply, or catabolic state
- Bleeding: abnormal vasculature in growing tumor, erosion of tumor into minor and major blood vessels, dry mucous membranes, GI disease (gastritis, varices, ulcers, inflammatory bowel); coagulopathy from chemotherapy, anticoagulation medication, hematologic cancers, or chronic disease
- Drainage: leakage of fluids from tumor vasculature, inflammatory processes due to infection, secretion of permeability factors by tumors, byproduct of bacterial proteases
- Malodor: byproducts of anaerobic and proteolytic bacteria growing in necrotic tissue

Findings

Biomedical

Malodorous and Draining Lesions

- Five percent to 10% of patients with cancer will develop a malignant wound.
- Most commonly found in breast, head and neck, and genital cancers
- Physically deforming fungating or ulcerating tumors
- Nonhealing decubitus or vascular ulcers
- Copious drainage, which may be odorless or malodorous
- Anorexia, nausea, fatigue, depression, altered sleep patterns, pruritus, reduced mobility, reduced activity
- Wound infection and cellulitis
- Pain due to dressing changes, pressure from tumor mass, erosion of lesion into tissues and nerves, exposure of dermal nerve endings, inflammation (see "Pain" later in this section)

Minor Bleeding

- Minor recurrent nosebleeds (epistaxis) or gingival bleeding caused by drying of mucous membranes or increased systolic BP

- Capillary oozing or other minor bleeding from open sores, decubiti, stomas, hemorrhoids, macerated/abraded skin (e.g., perineum, sacrum)
- Petechial bleeding due to thrombocytopenia

Moderate to Major Bleeding

- GI blood loss (melena, hematochezia, hematemesis)
- Genitourinary blood loss (hematuria, vaginal bleeding)
- Pulmonary blood loss (hemoptysis)
- Vigorous blood loss from mucous membranes, skin lesions, and stomas that have eroded major blood vessels
- Disruption of major blood vessels by necrosis or tumor
- Fatigue, dyspnea, tachycardia, hypotension
- Nausea, vomiting and diarrhea may be associated with swallowed blood or GI bleeding.
- Pain

Psychosocial/Spiritual

- Wounds can have a devastating impact on quality of life. Hospice staff should explore these potential psychosocial and spiritual findings with patients, caregivers and loved ones:
  - Fear of disease progression and anxiety over people seeing or smelling the wound
  - Panic from the thought of exsanguination or suffocation
  - Aesthetic anguish, embarrassment, humiliation, shame, stigmatization
  - Depression, anxiety, guilt, disgust, worthlessness, helplessness
  - Social isolation and withdrawal, avoidance, concealing
  - Loss of femininity, masculinity, sexuality, or intimacy
  - Loss of control

Assessment

Biomedical

Malodor and Drainage

- Determine source and quantity of drainage.
- Assess for infection: purulence, erythema, warmth, induration, fever, pain.
- Assess for pain (location, quality, severity, temporal relationships).

Bleeding

- Determine source of bleeding and examine specific site if possible.
- Inspect open wounds and dressings for evidence of bleeding.
- Determine rate and amount of bleeding.
- Determine likelihood of catastrophic hemorrhage (exsanguinating).
- Assess for signs and symptoms of blood loss anemia (fatigue, dyspnea, pallor).
- Assess patient and caregiver goals regarding bleeding, anemia, and transfusions.
- Check hemoglobin only if infusion of blood products is an appropriate palliative measure in the context of the patient's goals, preferences, and functional status.

Psychosocial/Spiritual

- Assess degree of distress caused by malodor and drainage.
- Elicit patient and caregiver fears about bleeding.
- Review or initiate discussions of advance directives with regard to massive blood loss.
- Identify any specific religious or other injunctions against the use of blood products.

Practical

- Identify readily accessible resources to deal with massive blood loss (see "hemorrhage kit" later in this topic).
- Determine caregiver knowledge and ability to manage wound care and dressing changes.

Processes of Care

Biomedical

Malodorous and Draining Lesions

- For cleansing use warm water, saline, or a mild wound-cleansing product.
- Debridement may be helpful for heavily necrotic wounds but is not recommended for fungating malignant wounds due to risk of bleeding and poor granulation potential.
- Dressings should be chosen for long length of wear, patient preference, and cost. The best dressings have a permeable nonadherent contact layer (such as foam or a soft silicon perforated sheet) with a secondary absorbent layer containing hydrogel (for mild drainage) or hydrocolloid (for moderate drainage). Alginate dressings are useful for absorbing heavy exudate and are nonadhesive if soaked with saline prior to removal.
- Other options for refractory malodorous wounds
  - Topical metronidazole (two 500-mg tabs crushed, or 0.75% gel or 1% cream) applied directly to wound or to dressing daily after wound care
  - Oral metronidazole (500 mg PO TID)
  - Activated charcoal dressings
  - Antimicrobial dressings

Infected Wounds

- Clinically infected wounds should be treated with systemic antibiotics if feasible and if consistent with patient preferences and goals.
- Avoid toxic antiseptic agents such as iodine, peroxide, Dakin's solution, and acetic acid as they can impair granulation. Iodine-containing antiseptic solutions may be helpful, however, in necrotic or gangrenous tissue to decrease bacterial burden.
- If antiseptic agents are needed due to wound infection and high bacterial burden of viable tissue, silver-impregnated dressings and cadexomer iodine have been shown to be less damaging. Irradiated medical-grade honey has also been used successfully to prevent bacterial growth.

Painful Cutaneous Lesions
- See "Pain" later in this section for use of systemic analgesics.
- Dressing removal is the greatest source of pain for patients with wounds:
  - Minimize dressing changes as much as possible and practical.
  - Use nonadherent contact dressings.
  - Moisten dry dressings prior to removal.
  - Premedicate with a short-acting opioid 30 minutes prior to wound care.
- EMLA 5% (eutectic mixture of local anesthetic) cream applied in a thick layer over a wound 30 minutes prior to debridement can significantly reduce pain.
- Topical lidocaine 2.75% in zinc oxide cream can provide up to 4 hours of local pain relief to fungating wounds.
- Topical morphine compounded 10 mg/ml in 8 g of Intrasite gel applied to painful ulcers and wounds one to three times daily and covered with Tegaderm dressing may be helpful for some patients.
- Aerosolized 0.5% bupivacaine or a paste of aluminum hydroxide/magnesium hydroxide may relieve burning and stinging.

Minor Bleeding: Topical Sites
- General principles
  - Minimize dressing changes to when blood is visible through dressings.
  - Moisten dressings with warm saline before removal.
  - Apply gentle pressure to minor bleeding for 10 minutes.
  - Similar dressing guidelines as management of drainage: a nonadherent layer combined with an absorptive dressing (soft silicones, hydrogels, petroleum gauze, and foam dressings are appropriate for absorbing small amounts of bleeding; alginate, sucralfate, and hydrocolloid dressings tend to be the most absorptive and hemostatic)
- Topical coagulant products
  - Silver Gelfoam sponge or powder to bleeding site. Follow package instructions carefully.
  - Silver nitrate sticks topically to bleeding site if well localized; hold stick to bleeding point followed by a gentle rotating motion.
  - Sucralfate paste, or sucralfate tabs 1 to 2 g crushed with water-soluble gel. Apply to wound one or two times daily.
  - Thromboplastin powder applied under dressings
- Topical vasoconstrictors
  - Oxymetazoline spray applied to wound prior to dressing
  - Topical epinephrine (1:1,000 = 1 mg/1 ml), dilute 1 ml in 100 ml normal saline (final solution of 1:100,000); apply to gauze and then apply with pressure for 10 minutes. Use with caution; may cause rebound bleeding and may aggravate necrosis.

Major Bleeding
- General principles
  - Identify patients at risk and have plans in place ahead of time (see "Psychosocial and Practical" below).
  - Apply pressure to bleeding site if accessible.

- Catastrophic hemorrhage usually results in death within minutes. Anxiolytic medications may be helpful for some patients but may also serve as a distraction to nurses and caregivers, whose primary focus should be to remain with the patient and remain calm. If anxiolytics are desired, diazepam 10 mg IM is the most expedient approach. If this is not practical, can also use lorazepam 4 mg SL (onset 5 minutes) or diazepam 10 mg rectal suppository (onset is 10 to 15 minutes).
- When the routine topical approaches listed above are not successful, not tolerated, or not practical, pharmacotherapy with fibrinolytic inhibitors may be indicated:
  - Tranexamic acid
    - 1.5 g PO loading dose followed by 1 g PO tid for internal bleeding
    - Dissolve 500 mg in 5 ml of saline and soak into gauze; apply with pressure for 10 minutes for mild oropharyngeal bleeding or other topical sites tid or prn.
    - 1 g dissolved in 10 ml saline swish-and-swallow tid for moderate to severe oropharyngeal bleeding
  - Aminocaproic acid
    - 5 g PO loading dose followed by 1 g PO qid
    - Same alternate dilutions and routes as tranexamic acid above
- Consider adjuvant therapies such as palliative radiation in anticipation of potential bleeding or after initial bleeding is controlled. Other adjuvant therapies include bronchoscopy, endoscopy, or cystoscopy for arterial embolization. Referrals should always be made with consideration of goals, comfort, life expectancy, and functional status.

Specific Bleeding Sites
- In addition to the above general guidelines for topical and systemic treatment of bleeding, the following are special considerations for specific bleeding sites:
  - Nasopharyngeal bleeding (epistaxis)
    - Avoid disruption of crusted scabs in nose.
    - Keep patient in high-Fowler position with head slightly bent forward.
    - Provide constant pressure to outer nares for 5 to 10 minutes.
    - Apply cold compresses to nape of neck.
    - Provide cool mist humidification to room air or to nasal cannula to reduce drying of nasal passages.
    - Oxymetazoline nasal spray up to qid: DO NOT BLOW NOSE AFTER SPRAY.
    - Silver nitrate stick if bleeding site can be visualized
  - Oropharyngeal bleeding
    - Epinephrine-soaked gauze
    - Topical or swish-and-swallow fibrinolytic inhibitor
    - Sucralfate suspension mouthwash (1 g dissolved in 10 ml water bid)
  - Hemoptysis
    - Consider benefits and burdens of ruling out pulmonary embolism prior to administering fibrinolytic inhibitor.
    - Consider oral dexamethasone 4 mg PO daily.

- Upper GI bleeding
  - Proton pump inhibitor
  - Oral fibrinolytic inhibitor
  - Oral sucralfate 2 g PO bid
  - Consider IV/SQ octreotide.
- Lower GI bleeding
  - Oral fibrinolytic inhibitor
  - Rectal sucralfate (2 g mixed into aqueous jelly bid)
  - Tranexamic acid enema (5 g dissolved into 50 ml warm water bid)
- Urinary tract bleeding
  - Consider inserting Foley catheter to prevent outflow obstruction from clots.
  - Irrigate Foley catheter with normal saline to maintain patency if concern for obstruction.
  - Use fibrinolytic inhibitors with caution as they may cause clotting.
  - Cover urinary drainage bag in presence of gross hematuria.

Psychosocial and Practical

- For nonhealing wounds, help redirect goals away from healing and more toward comfort, keeping the wound clean, and preventing infection.
- In the event of a major bleeding episode, *stay with the patient and family*. Catastrophic hemorrhage typically results in loss of consciousness within minutes, and death shortly thereafter. The most important thing the family is likely to remember was the calm presence of hospice staff.
- Identify patients potentially at risk for major bleeding and educate them and their families about what to expect. Elicit their wishes and fears in the event of major bleeding.
- Instruct families to call hospice in the event of bleeding.
- Explain in advance the options for crisis care or general inpatient hospice placement based on family preferences and ability to cope with major bleeding.
- Advise families to prepare a "hemorrhage kit," which should contain dressing supplies, gloves, dark towels and washcloths, absorbent blue pads (Chux), plastic mattress cover, black garbage bags.
- Educate caregivers to remove and replace soiled dressings, clothes, sheets, and towels as soon as possible.
- Instruct caregivers on universal precautions and handling of bodily fluids (see "Basic Home Safety" in Section 2).
- Inform caregivers that bleeding episodes may be accompanied by symptoms of anxiety, restlessness, cool moist skin, and increased pallor.

Goals/Outcomes

- Minimize emotional distress and social isolation
- Reduce or stop bleeding from all sites to the extent possible
- Prevent caregiver avoidance of patient
- Anticipate and treat painful wounds with appropriate analgesics

- Facilitate reasoned self-determination about various approaches to therapy for symptomatic blood loss, especially in the consideration of palliative transfusion
- Prevent panic in the event of major bleeding

Documentation in the Medical Record

Initial Medical and Psychosocial Assessment

- Causes and severity of malodorous lesions or bleeding
- Patient/caregiver reactions to malodorous lesions or bleeding
- Likelihood of hemorrhagic event
- Symptoms/signs of anemia

Interdisciplinary Progress Notes

- Content of discussions with patient, family, and caregivers
- Results of wound-care interventions

IDT Care Plan

- Detailed wound-care plan
- Frequency of nursing visits for wound care
- Contingency plan in event of major bleeding

Recommended Reading

Adderly UJ, Holt IG. Topical agents and dressings for fungating wounds. *Cochrane Database Syst Rev* 2014; 5:CD003948.

Alexander S. Malignant fungating wounds: key symptoms and psychosocial issues. *J Wound Care* 2009; 18(8):325–329.Association for the Advancement of Wound Care (AAWC). *Pressure ulcer guidelines*. Malvern, PA: AAWC, 2010. Available at http://aawconline.org/wpcontent/uploads/2011/08/AAWCPressureUlcerGuidelineofGuidelinesAug11.pdf.

Chrisman C. Care of chronic wounds in palliative care and end-of-life patients. *Intl Wound J* 2010; 7(4):214–235.

Da Costo Santos C, Pimenta C, Nobre MA. Systematic review of topical treatments to control the odor of malignant fungating wounds. *J Pain Symptom Manage* 2010; 39(6):1065–1076.

Gibson S, Green J. Review of patients' experiences with fungating wounds and associated quality of life. *J Wound Care* 2013; 22(5):265–275.

Harris DG, Finlay IG, Flowers S, Noble SIR. The use of crisis medication in the management of terminal haemorrhage due to incurable cancer: a qualitative study. *Palliat Med* 2011; 25:691–700.

Hulme B, Wilcox S. *Guidelines on the management of bleeding for palliative care patients with cancer*. Yorkshire Palliative Medicine Clinical Guidelines Group. November 2008. Available at www.palliativedrugs.com/download/090331_Final_bleeding_guidelines.pdf.

LaBon B, Zeppetella G Higginson I. Effectiveness of topical administration of opioids in palliative care: a systematic review. *J Pain Symptom Manage* 2009; 37(5):913–917.

Lo SF, Hayter M, Hu WY, et al. Symptom burden and quality of life in patients with malignant fungating wounds. *J Adv Nurs* 2012; 68(6):1312–1321.

Recka K, Montagnini M, Vitale C. Management of bleeding associated with malignant wounds. *J Palliat Med* 2012; 15(8):952–952.

Wodash AJ. Wet-to-dry dressings do not provide moist wound healing. *J Am Coll Clin Wound Spec* 2012; 4(3):63–66.

Confusion/Delirium

SITUATION: Change in mental status with acute confusion that interferes with ability to carry out activities of daily living and maintain patient safety and adds to caregiver burden.

Causes

Biomedical

- Systemic infection (e.g., common occurrence in the elderly with urinary tract infection, pneumonia)
- Dehydration
- Toxic drug reactions (common occurrences due to anticholinergic drugs or anticholinergic effects from many drug classes, or other CNS cognitive adverse effects from antidepressants, benzodiazepines, corticosteroids, antiemetics, sedatives, opioids, anticonvulsants)
- Opioids are commonly used in palliative care, and their neuropsychiatric side effects, often collectively referred to as opioid-induced neurotoxicity, commonly occur in patients with advanced diseases.
- Organic brain syndrome from underlying disease (e.g., primary brain or metastatic cancer, AIDS dementia, hydrocephalus, degenerative brain changes, cerebrovascular occlusion or bleeding, post-radiation therapy for brain neoplasm[s])
- Metabolic or physiologic derangement (e.g., hypercalcemia; hyponatremia; hyper- or hypoglycemia; electrolyte imbalance; uremia; thyroid dysfunction; adrenal disease; advanced liver, renal, or respiratory impairment; fecal impaction; urinary retention; urinary tract infection)
- Acute abstinence syndrome (alcohol, opioids, benzodiazepines, psychoactive drugs)
- Undertreated pain

Psychosocial/Spiritual

- Psychological decompensation from social stressors
- Depression ("pseudo-dementia")
- Expressions of fear, uncertainty, unpreparedness, unfinished business, and emotional unrest
- Pathological grief reaction in anticipation of loss
- Environmental
- Hospitalization/ICU disorientation
- Sleep deprivation
- Psychological stress from noxious procedures (e.g., urethral catheterization)
- Communication impairment

Findings

Biomedical

- Stigmata of coexisting disease to be found during systemic review and physical examination
- Decreased or increased level of activity (i.e., somnolent vs. restless/agitated)

Psychosocial

- Alterations in perception and cognition (i.e., decreased or fluctuating level of consciousness, disorientation, and misperception); may become evident only after a long discussion or several visits with the patient

Assessment

Biomedical

- Review medications for drugs that may cause or contribute to confusion, especially recently added psychotropic agents or changes in drug or dosing schedule.
- Collect data from family or caregivers regarding patient's mental status before the onset of delirium.
- Assess for metabolic derangement based on likelihoods (e.g., blood sugar abnormalities in a known diabetic).
- Associated signs and symptoms
  - Uremia: oliguria/anuria; "frost" on facial skin
  - Hyperglycemia: polydipsia, polyuria, blurred vision, "fruity" odor to breath
  - Hypoglycemia: lethargy to unarousability, tachycardia, diaphoresis
  - Hypercalcemia: polydipsia, polyuria, nausea, ileus, muscle twitching
- Determine relative burdens (intrusiveness and costs of tests) versus benefits (likelihood of improvement from specific therapeutic interventions) in concert with patient/family goals.
- Assess for presence of fever or common sources of infection: urinary, respiratory, skin (pressure sores, abscess, cellulitis).
- Assess for signs of neurologic change to suggest brain metastasis:
  - Volatile mood/behavior or fluctuating level of consciousness, hallucinations, thought disorder
  - Headache
  - Nausea/vomiting
  - Visual impairment (double vision; field cut)
  - Motor, sensory, coordination alteration or deficit
  - Papilledema
- Assess for withdrawal symptoms from alcohol or other drugs:
  - Time of last dose or drink
  - Tachycardia, tachypnea, diaphoresis, hypertension
  - Nausea, abdominal pain, diarrhea
  - Pupillary dilatation (mydriasis)
  - Restlessness, hallucinations, paranoia

Psychosocial

- Perform Mini-Mental Status Examination (compare with previous baseline if available):
  - Orientation (person, place, time, situation)
  - Remote and recent memory (last four presidents, children's/grandchildren's names/birthdates, ability to recall four items after 5 to 10 minutes)
  - Cognitive function (ability to read simple text and comprehend it; ability to subtract serial 7s from 100; ability to tell time)

- Reasoning (what would you do if you smelled smoke in the house?)
- Abstraction (what does "people who live in glass houses shouldn't throw stones" mean?)
- Spatial integrity (draw a round clock face with numbers and hands)
- Assess for presence of insomnia.
- Assess for presence of delusions and/or hallucinations.
- Other assessment tools include:
  - Confusion Assessment Method (CAM; see http://consultgerirn.org/uploads/File/trythis/try_this_13.pdf); CAM should not replace clinical judgment in the diagnosis of delirium
  - Memorial Delirium Assessment Scale (MDAS; see http://crashingpatient.com/wp-content/pdf/MDAS.pdf)
  - Short Orientation Memory Concentration Test
  - Nurse Delirium Screening Scale
  - Newer tools that are promising but will require further validation include 4AT, Months of Years Backwards, Delirium Observational Screening Scale, Observational Scale of Level of Arousal.

Processes of Care

Practical

- Instruct caregiver(s) on reality orientation (frequent reminders of time and place; provide cues such as large-numbered calendar and clock).
- Allay fear: use visual and hearing aids.
- Instruct caregiver(s) on need for simple, structured routine and quiet, calm environment as much as possible.
- Provide interventions to ensure adequate periods of rest.
- "Routine-ize" defecation/urination (for continent patients), nutrition, mobilization.
  - Avoid physical restraints.
  - Normalize sleep–wake cycle.

Biomedical

- Medicate according to need for patient safety, to relieve distressing symptoms, and to obtain reasonable periods of rest, per physician orders.
  - Management is largely guided by expert opinion and consensus-based clinical guidelines.
  - There is no convincing evidence to suggest that any one drug class is superior to another.
- Notify attending physician if assessment indicates an etiology that is new or imminently treatable.
- Pharmacotherapy for palliation of delirium/agitation unrelieved by primary therapies or milieu therapy (*NOTE: No medications have been approved by the U.S. Food and Drug Administration [FDA] with specific indications for the treatment of delirium*)
  1. Haloperidol 1 to 2 mg orally q2–4hr prn. In the elderly, start at a lower dose of 0.25 to 0.5 mg to minimize adverse effects and side effects. Haloperidol can be given orally, via feeding tubes, IV, SQ, or IM. Titrate upward as needed.

2. Benzodiazepines are not routinely used unless delirium is caused by benzodiazepine or alcohol withdrawal or is related to seizures. Benzodiazepines may have a limited role in addition to an antipsychotic but should be avoided as single agents in the treatment of delirium.
3. Chlorpromazine (25 mg PO/PR q6–8hr) is an acceptable alternative to haloperidol if greater sedation is desirable.
4. Atypical antipsychotics (risperidone 0.5 to 1 mg bid, olanzapine 2.5 to 5 mg/day, quetiapine 50 to 100 mg bid) are alternatives in managing delirium. The FDA has issued a black-box warning of increased risk of death when these antipsychotics are used to treat elderly patients with dementia-related psychoses.
5. Follow guidelines in "Agitation and Anxiety" earlier in this section if confusional state progresses to a more severe state of agitation.
   - Opioid-induced neurotoxicity is managed by opioid rotation or switching and/or dose reduction.
   - All cholinesterase inhibitors (e.g., donepezil, rivastigmine, galantamine) should be avoided in the treatment or prevention of delirium.
   - The role of melatonin in reducing delirium in palliative care patients warrants further study.

Psychosocial

- Provide a quiet environment: reduce unnecessary noise, activity, clutter, excessive light, excessive darkness.
- Speak clearly in simple short sentences; avoid complex explanations; be sure patient can hear you.
- Direct patient's attention on the present.
- Identify and focus on patient's strengths.
- Involve social worker early to assist patient and caregiver with coping skills and to identify need for volunteers and other expertise within the IDT.
- Provide support to caregiver.
  - Anticipate cognitive changes with disease progression and educate caregivers to report early, potentially reversible alternations in mental status.
  - Believe caregiver's observations about changes in patient's mental state (these may be subtle to outside observers who see the patient on an occasional basis only).
  - Arrange for volunteer to relieve family.
  - Assist family to schedule rest periods so that someone is resting when another is with the patient.
  - Allow caregiver to voice concerns, sadness, and/or anger regarding change in patient's personality.

Goals/Outcomes

- Patient is able to rest comfortably without excessive fear, agitation, or restlessness.
  - If delirium resolves, a trial of discontinuation of drug therapy used for treatment should be considered, especially if a primary etiology is identified and treated or reversed.
  - Debriefing for patients who have recovered from an episode of delirium

- Maximize patient's ability to communicate needs and express feelings.
- Caregiver burden is minimized to allow adequate periods of rest and sleep and uninterrupted household activities.
- Safe environment is provided for patient and caregiver.
- Prevent unnecessary transfers

Documentation in the Medical Record

Initial Medical Assessment

- Precipitating factors leading to confusion
- Signs and symptoms of concurrent or progressive disease
- Findings from systems review and physical examination
- Differential diagnosis of etiology of acute signs/symptoms

Initial Psychosocial Assessment

- Patient behaviors and results of mental status examination
- Goals of therapy and advance directives reviewed/discussed

Interdisciplinary Progress Notes

- Results of interventions
- Observations from repeated assessments
- Caregiver coping

IDT Care Plan

- Order of evaluation and treatment approaches
- Specific interventions
- Contingency plans

Recommended Reading

Bush SH, Bruera E, Lawlor PG, et al. Clinical practice guidelines for delirium management: potential application in palliative care. *J Pain Symptom Manage* 2014; 48(2):249–258.

Leonard MM, Nekolaichuk C, Meagher DJ, et al. Practical assessment of delirium in palliative care. *J Pain Symptom Manage* 2014; 48(2):176–190.

Rao S, Ferris FD, Irwin SA. Ease of screening for depression and delirium in patients enrolled in inpatient hospice care. *J Palliat Med* 2011; 14(3):275–279.

Wright DK, Brajtmann S. A relational ethical approach to end-of-life delirium. *J Pain Symptom Manage* 2014; 48(2):191–197.

Constipation

SITUATION: Decreased bowel motility with consequent constipation, distention, obstipation, or impaction.

Causes

- Decreased autonomic function due to aging
- Decreased activity

- Alterations in food and fluid intake
- Inaccessibility of toilet due to decreased mobility, sedation, etc., leading to retention of stool
- Pharmacological effects of opioid analgesics and drugs with anticholinergic activity (e.g., tricyclic antidepressants)
- Painful anorectal lesions (e.g., hemorrhoids, fissures) leading to retention of stool
- Weakness due to primary disease or secondary to asthenia
- Hypokalemia; hypercalcemia

Findings

- Patient report or caregiver assessment of decreased bowel movement frequency, hard stool, or painful elimination
- Soiling of clothing due to seepage of liquid stool around impacted stool in rectum
- Sense of bloating with abdominal distention
- Increase or absence of bowel sounds
- No bowel movement for at least 2 days
- Painful anal lesions

Assessment

- Bowel assessment should be a regular part of every patient visit. Consider use of a constipation assessment scale such as the Constipation Assessment Scale or the Constipation Visual Analogue Scale (see http://www.thefreelibrary.com/Modified+Constipation+Assessment+Scale+is+an+effective+tool+to+assess...-a0138224937).
- Determine date of last bowel movement and stool characteristics.
- Review 24-hour food and fluid intake.
- Determine patient's ability to respond to urge to defecate (generate adequate bearing down).
- Determine patient's ability to get to toilet or notify caregiver for help in toileting.
- Auscultate and examine abdomen for quality and intensity (or absence) of bowel sounds, masses, and tenderness.
- Observe, percuss, and palpate abdomen for distention, tympany, and tenderness.
- Assess for and rule out urinary retention commonly associated with fecal impaction.
- Determine if new-onset nausea/vomiting is present, suspicious for bowel obstruction.
- Perform an anorectal examination for lesions, muscle tone, retained stool, impaction.

Processes of Care

Practical and Biomedical

- Notify physician if evidence of bowel obstruction.
- Convenience (access to facilities), comfort, and privacy (dignity) should be optimized to promote regular bowel movements and prevent retention.

- All patients taking opioid analgesics should be on some form of anticonstipation regimen.
- Increase hydration if consistent with patient wishes and if benefits would likely outweigh burdens.
- Never use motility agents when there are signs or symptoms of bowel obstruction.
- Disimpaction and enemas should precede use of motility agents.
- Recommend or allow use of psyllium (e.g., Metamucil) or bulking foods and fiber (fruits, bran, etc.) in active and well-hydrated patients only.
- Pharmacotherapy for constipation
  - Rectal suppositories should be placed up against wall of the rectum, not in substance of stool.
  - Glycerin suppositories for dry, hard, difficult-to-pass stool
  - Starting anticonstipation regimen
    — Senna preparation (e.g., Senokot tabs one or two tabs PO at HS, and increase up to four tabs tid [may substitute 5 ml of liquid Senokot for each tablet]) as needed; or
    — Bisacodyl 5 mg, one or two tablets PO at HS or bisacodyl 10 mg suppository PR at HS; double, then triple the dose, adding morning and afternoon doses
  - If no bowel movement within 24 to 48 hours, for hard, desiccated stool, add a stool softener (e.g., docusate sodium 250 mg qd to bid).
  - If no bowel movement within 48 hours of initiating therapy, use phosphate (Fleet) enema.
- If no bowel movement within 72 hours of initiating therapy, repeat rectal examination; if no evidence of bowel obstruction, no impaction, and no result from oil retention enema (4 oz warmed mineral oil or Fleet Mineral Oil Enema) followed by phosphate enema:
  - Magnesium citrate 8 oz PO or mineral oil 30 to 60 ml PO
  - Lactulose 10 to 30 ml PO qd or bid
- Peripheral opioid antagonist therapy
  - Methylnaltrexone is a peripherally acting mu-opioid receptor antagonist with restricted ability to cross the blood–brain barrier; it reverses opioid-induced constipation without affecting analgesia.
  - The recommended dose of the approved injectable form of methylnaltrexone is 8 mg for patients weighing 38 to 62 kg (84 to 136 lb) or 12 mg for patients weighing 62 to 114 kg (136 to 251 lb); patients whose weight falls outside of these ranges should be dosed at 0.15 mg/kg.
  - Studies have reported that between 48% and 62% of patients treated with methylnaltrexone have a bowel movement within 4 hours of SQ administration; ensure that there is no impaction before administration.
  - Naloxegol is an oral agent that blocks mu-opioid receptor activation in the intestinal tract.
    - Available in doses of 12.5 mg and 25 mg
    - Recommendations for use
      a. Discontinue all other laxatives prior to use.
      b. Start with 25 mg, but reduce to 12.5 mg if the higher dose is not tolerated; for patients with renal impairment, start with 12.5 mg.

    c. Take on an empty stomach at least 1 hour prior to the first meal of the day.
    d. Avoid grapefruit, grapefruit juice, and other CYP3A4 inhibitors.
- Manual disimpaction
  - Apply local anesthetic preparation (e.g., EMLA cream, lidocaine 2% ointment or 4% gel) liberally to external and internal anal mucosa and administer 4 oz of warm mineral oil into rectal vault 15 to 30 minutes prior to digital dilatation and stool removal.
  - If this process causes distress, especially when repeat disimpaction is required, premedication with lorazepam 1 to 2 mg and the patient's usual breakthrough dose of analgesic 30 to 60 minutes before manual disimpaction will usually produce favorable conditions.

Goals/Outcomes

- Painless, regular bowel movements at least every 3 days
- Absence of induced diarrhea and abdominal cramping from bowel regimen
- Confidence in use of opioid analgesics for pain relief without worry over bowel function

Documentation in the Medical Record

Admission Assessment

- Review of bowel function
- Risks of impending bowel dysfunction due to disease, medications, activity, food/fluid intake
- Patient's and/or family caregiver's ability to manage own bowel care

Physical Examination Findings

Medication Review

Dietary Assessment

Interdisciplinary Progress Notes

- History of bowel actions and toileting ability
- Use of bowel protocol
- Therapeutic and adverse effects of bowel protocol
- Findings from repeated physical examination

IDT Care Plan

- Progressive implementation of bowel protocol
- Instructions to patient/caregiver
- Schedule of follow-up evaluations of adherence to bowel protocol and reassessments

Recommended Reading

Argoff CE, Brennan MJ, Camilleri M, et al. Consensus recommendations on initiating prescription therapies for opioid-induced constipation. *Pain Med* 2015; 16(12):2324–2337.

Larkin PJ, Sykes NP, Centeno C, et al; European Consensus Group on Constipation in Palliative Care. The management of constipation in palliative care: clinical practice recommendations. *Palliat Med* 2008; 22(7):796–807.

Naloxegol for opioid-induced constipation. *JAMA* 2016; 315(2):194–195.

Rauck RL. Treatment of opioid-induced constipation: focus on the peripheral μ-opioid receptor antagonist methylnaltrexone. *Drugs* 2013; 73(12):1297–1306.

Weber HC. Opioid-induced constipation in chronic noncancer pain. *Curr Opin Endocrinol Diabetes Obes* 2016; 23(1):11–17.

Coughing

SITUATION: Frequent cough with resultant pain or discomfort, inability to rest, social disruption, sleep disruption, risk of rib fracture.

Causes

- Pulmonary infection
- COPD and other chronic lung diseases
- Decreased mobility
- Weakness with reduced effectiveness of cough (ineffective clearing of airways)
- Sinus infection
- Respiratory system neoplasm
- Pulmonary edema
- Pleural effusion
- Reactive airways disease (asthma)
- Heart failure
- Gastroesophageal reflux disease
- ACE inhibitors
- Environmental irritants and allergies

Findings

- Loose, productive cough
- Dry, nonproductive cough
- Exasperation, exhaustion, chest pain

Assessment

Practical

- Check for potential sources of airway irritation (dust, allergenic pillows, pet dander, blooming plants, etc.).

Biomedical

- History of new-onset versus recurrent versus chronic cough
- Review history of smoking, asthma, occupational factors.
- Obtain history of triggering and relieving factors.
- Medication review

- Assess cough (frequency, quality, intensity, muscle power, nocturnal or daytime).
- Assess sputum characteristics (volume, color, purulence).
- Auscultate lungs for adventitious breath sounds (rhonchi, rales, wheezes), diminished breath sounds, pleural rub.
- Check for peripheral edema, jugular venous distention, gallop rhythm.
- Rule out associated paroxysmal nocturnal dyspnea or orthopnea.
- Check for use of accessory muscles of respiration, tachypnea, tachycardia, cyanosis.
- Assess for fever.
- Check for sinus tenderness, nasal discharge.

Psychosocial

- Assess impact of cough on mood, sleep, energy, pain, social interaction.

Processes of Care

Biomedical

- Treat specific etiology of cough if identified (e.g., antibiotics, nonsedating antihistamines, diuretics, bronchodilators).
- If central airway obstruction, consider palliative chemotherapy, palliative radiotherapy, endobronchial laser resection, or stent placement (if concordant with goals of care and prognosis).
- Instruct in proper use of nebulizer, if indicated.
- Aggressively treat symptoms in concert with the degree of distress being caused.
- Increase humidity in patient's environment—cool mist vaporizer in room.
- Elevate head of bed.
- Chest physical therapy
- Palliative pharmacotherapy
  - Nebulized saline
  - Expectorants
    — Guaifenesin 5 ml PO q4hr prn or one or two tablets PO q12hr up to four tablets/24 hr
  - Centrally acting antitussives
    - OTC dextromethorphan-containing cough syrup: use as directed (usually 1 to 2 tsp PO q4hr)
    - Codeine 15 to 30 mg PO q4hr prn (*NOTE: Adjust dose based on other opioid analgesic use and institute constipation prevention/treatment care plan*)
  - Peripherally acting antitussives
    - Benzonatate 100 to 200 mg PO tid
  - Treat insomnia if nocturnal cough unabated by above therapies (refer to "Insomnia and Nocturnal Restlessness" later in this section).
  - Nebulized opioids and local anesthetics
  - Opioid receptors are expressed in bronchopulmonary tissues with great variability.
  - Consider nebulized opioids or lidocaine in severe, refractory cases (data mixed on efficacy; no high-quality data exist).

- Initial opioid dosing: morphine 5 mg/2 ml in 0.9% saline or fentanyl 25 mcg/2 ml in saline (fentanyl, being more lipophilic and less allergenic, may be advantageous)
- Initial local anesthetic dosing: lidocaine 5 ml of 2% solution (cautious titration and frequency of dosing due to variable absorption and risk of systemic toxicity)
- Corticosteroids
  - Dexamethasone 4 to 12 mg PO daily
- Instruct in appropriate handling and disposal of sputum (refer to "Basic Home Safety" in Section 2).

Goals/Outcomes

- Ability to clear airways and expectorate sputum and bronchopulmonary secretions
- Reduce coughing paroxysms to the extent possible based on the underlying disease
- Increase periods of rest and uninterrupted sleep
- Improve social interaction
- Maximize hygiene
- Prevent and treat cough-related pain

Documentation in the Medical Record

Initial Assessment

- Findings of cardiopulmonary systems review and physical examination
- Impact of cough on patient/caregiver

Interdisciplinary Progress Notes

- Results of interventions and ongoing assessments

IDT Care Plan

- Specific interventions and associated goals
- Follow-up and contingency plans

Recommended Reading

Hayes D, Anstead M, Warner R, et al. Inhaled morphine for palliation of dyspnea in end-stage cystic fibrosis. *Am J Health-System Pharmacy* 2010; 67(9):737–740.

Lv ZM, Chen L, Tang J. Nebulized lidocaine inhalation in the treatment of patients with acute asthma. *World J Emerg Med* 2011; 2(1):30–32.

Molassiotis A, Bailey C, Caress A, Tan JY. Interventions for cough in cancer. *Cochrane Database Syst Rev* 2015; 5:CD007881.

Molassiotis A, Smith J, Bennett M, et al. Clinical expert guidelines for the management of cough in lung cancer: report of a UK task group on cough. *Cough* 2010; 6:9.

Simoff MJ, Lally B, Slade MG, et al. Symptom management in patients with lung cancer: diagnosis and management of lung cancer. Third edition of American College of Chest Physicians evidence-based clinical practice guidelines. *Chest* 2013; 143:e455S.

Truesdale K, Jurdi A. Nebulized lidocaine in the treatment of intractable cough. *Am J Hosp Palliat Care* 2013; 30:587.

Wee B, Browning J, Adams A, et al. Management of chronic cough in patients receiving palliative care: review of evidence and recommendations by a task group of the Association for Palliative Medicine of Great Britain and Ireland. *Palliat Med* 2012; 26:780.

Depression

SITUATION: Depressed mood or unexplained poor adherence to treatment that interferes with patient care or ability to cope with the dying process

Causes (Risk Factors)

Biomedical

- History of clinical depression or mental illness
- Terminal disease
- Uncontrolled distressing symptoms, particularly pain
- Sleep disorder
- Neurologic involvement of disease (e.g., primary or metastatic CNS tumors or AIDS)
- Adverse effect of certain medications (e.g., glucocorticoids) or general medical condition causing depression (e.g., hypercalcemia or hypothyroidism)
- Family history of depressive disorders

Psychosocial/Spiritual

- Poor spiritual support
- Existential concerns: loss of function, self-image, future, crisis of faith, etc.
- Boredom, social isolation, sense of uselessness/purposelessness/meaninglessness, lack of goals

Findings (Symptoms)

Biomedical

- Sleep disturbance or insomnia
- Expression of uncontrolled pain or other distressing symptoms (e.g., nausea, chronic cough, etc.) out of proportion to expected course of the patient's individual disease
- Impaired capacity for pleasure or decreased interest in enjoyable activities
- Inappropriate medication/substance use or frank misuse of mood-altering agents (alcohol, illicit drugs, analgesics, sedative–hypnotics)

Psychosocial/Spiritual

- Verbal or facial expression of sadness or depressed appearance, flat affect
- Social withdrawal, voluntary isolation

- "Vegetative signs" (e.g., hypersomnolence, decreased appetite, psychomotor retardation) may be suggestive but are not often used as sole criteria for diagnosis due to large amount of overlap with common symptoms of many terminal diseases.
- Volatile affect with agitation, anger, or crying
- Feelings of self-deprecation, guilt, hopelessness, helplessness that seem out of proportion to the patient's actual situation
- Passive or active suicidal ideation (e.g., "Everything would be better if I were dead" or "I don't deserve to live" or "I'm going to kill myself")
- Decreased adherence to palliative treatment or unexplainable difficulty managing disease symptoms

Assessment

Biomedical

- Determine role of underlying disease or uncontrolled symptoms as risk factors for depression.
- Evaluate effect of medications on signs and symptoms of depression.

Psychosocial/Spiritual

- Directly ask the question: "Have you felt depressed more days than not in the last few weeks?"
- Review past psychiatric history and response to loss or difficult life events.
- Understand patient/caregiver's perception of situation.
- Evaluate the effects of social factors on the symptoms of depression.
- Identify patient/caregiver's understanding of mental illness and capacity to address depression.
- Assess severity of depression, assess for the presence of suicidal thoughts and potential methods of suicide, and make an appropriate safety plan (refer to "Suicide: Risk, Prevention, Coping When It Happens" in Section 2). Ask about the presence of guns in the home if appropriate.
- Assess impact of depression on caregivers and their ability to cope.
- Facilitate discussion surrounding faith, values, definitions of hope and meaningfulness to determine potential role of spiritual crisis on depression symptoms.

Processes of Care

Biomedical

- Consult with physician regarding possible contributory medical conditions and adjustments; priority should be given to addressing uncontrolled symptoms and treating any reversible contributory general medical conditions or disruptions in sleep.
- Discuss indications for antidepressant pharmacotherapy during IDT review.
- Pharmacotherapy for treatment of depression

NOTE: Supportive counseling and empathic listening by members of the IDT (RN, social worker, chaplain, aide[s], physician, volunteers) should always complement pharmacotherapy. Selection of antidepressant medications should be based on symptoms, safety, simplicity of dosing, rapidity of response based on prognosis, safety profile, burden of adverse/side effects, and cost. Always monitor for metabolic disturbances and drug interactions that can lead to central serotonin toxicity.

1. Psychostimulants (e.g., methylphenidate, dextroamphetamine): Generally have more rapid onset of action than SSRIs and tricyclic or tetracyclic antidepressants (TCAs); helpful for patients with life expectancy less than 2 to 4 months. Methylphenidate starting dose is 2.5 or 5 mg PO every morning or every morning and midday; titrate up by 2.5 or 5 mg per dose for effect. Daily maximum 20 to 40 mg. Do not administer psychostimulant medications within 8 hours of anticipated bedtime.

2. SSRIs (e.g., fluoxetine, paroxetine, sertraline, citalopram, escitalopram): Generally preferred for starting treatment of depression, although they may take weeks for onset of action. May have significant drug interactions due to hepatic enzyme inhibition. Liquid formulations can be specially ordered.

   a. Fluoxetine: Starting dose is 10 or 20 mg PO daily; titrate up by 20 mg every 4 weeks for effect. Daily maximum 80 mg. Can switch to weekly formulation after symptom stabilization.

   b. Paroxetine: Starting dose is 10 or 20 mg PO every morning; titrate up by 10 mg every 7 days for effect. Daily maximum 50 mg.

   c. Sertraline: Starting dose is 50 mg PO daily; titrate up by 50 mg every 7 days for effect. Daily maximum 200 mg.

   d. Citalopram: Starting dose is 10 to 20 mg PO daily. Daily maximum is 20 mg in older patients due to increased risk of QT prolongation at higher doses.

   e. Escitalopram: Starting and maximum dose of 10 mg PO daily, due to risk of QT prolongation at higher doses.

3. TCAs (e.g., desipramine, nortriptyline, amitriptyline): Often useful for patients with insomnia or neuropathic pain, but limited use due to anticholinergic side effects. Liquid formulations are available for doxepin and nortriptyline.

   a. Nortriptyline: Starting dose for depression is 25 mg PO three or four times daily; titrate up to daily maximum 150 mg. Dosing can be switched to once daily after symptom stabilization.

4. Atypical antidepressants (e.g., mirtazapine, bupropion): Mirtazapine is found to be helpful in patients with insomnia, although it is less sedating at higher doses. Bupropion is helpful for patients with vegetative symptoms but often avoided in patients with severe illness due to its association with seizures.

   a. Mirtazapine: Starting dose for insomnia or depression is 7.5 or 15 mg PO q HS; titrate by 15 mg every 7 days as needed for depression. Daily maximum 45 mg.

5. SNRIs (e.g., venlafaxine, duloxetine)

   a. Venlafaxine: Starting dose for depression is 37.5 mg PO once or twice daily; titrate by 37.5 or 75 mg every 4 to 7 days for effect. Daily maximum 375 mg.

6. Serotonin modulators (e.g., trazodone, nefazodone, vilazodone)

   a. Trazodone: Starting dose for off-label use for insomnia is 50 mg PO q HS; titrate up by 50 mg as needed for effect. Starting dose for depression is 50 mg PO tid; titrate every 3 to 5 days as needed for effect. Daily maximum 400 mg.

Psychosocial/Spiritual

- Initiate discussion and promote expression of thoughts and feelings.
- Facilitate discussion of losses.
- Identify and reflect distortions in thinking; consider cognitive therapy.
- Help patient/caregiver identify and accept limits imposed by illness and assuage frustration of trying to control the uncontrollable.
- Help patient/caregiver identify what areas in their lives are still under their control and identify attainable goals.
- Engage patient/caregiver in life review; consider "dignity therapy."
- Identify and facilitate social interactions and recreational/distracting activities that may give meaning to daily life and minimize isolating behaviors.
- Determine if any foods give pleasure (regardless of nutritional value) and make available if possible.
- Determine patient's need to search for meaning in the dying experience and help him/her to find the language to express this; consider "meaning-centered therapy."
- Understand patient's values and preferences and facilitate these choices during the dying process to the extent possible.
- Help patient/caregiver to identify and use positive coping skills.
- Seek out and defer to expert medical/psychiatric treatment if signs/symptoms of depression do not respond to first-line approaches, if there is uncertainty about the psychiatric diagnosis, or if risk of suicide is significant.

Goals/Outcomes

- Reduce "vegetative" signs and symptoms
- Patient/caregiver will be able to express feelings of loss.
- Patient/caregiver will identify strategies to address depression symptoms.
- Patient/caregiver will report improved sense of well-being and ability to cope.
- Patient/caregiver will address issues raised by the level of debility, and potential insights imposed by progressive disease and foreseeable death will allow the opportunity for personal growth and finding value in the remaining days of life.

Documentation in the Medical Record

Initial Assessment

- Description of mood, sleep, activity, patient short-term goals (if any), patient's identified reasons for stated mood, presence of suicidal thoughts
- Patient's self-rating of depression (e.g., 0-to-5 scale: 0 = "Good mood; I do not feel sad or depressed at all" and 5 = "My mood is as low as it could possibly be. I find no meaning in my life.")

Interdisciplinary Progress Notes

- Description of interventions and results
- Repeat patient self-reports of depression scores (0-to-5 scale).

- Patient short-term (daily/weekly) attainable goals and results
- Follow up suicide risk.

IDT Care Plan

- Interventions planned
- Means to help patient attain stated goals
- Schedule of IDT visits

Recommended Reading

Breitbart W, Dickerman A. Assessment and management of depression in palliative care. In Roy-Byrne P, Block S, eds. *UpToDate*, 2015. Available at http://
www.uptodate.com/home/index.html.

Fitzgerald P, Miller K, Li M, Rodin G. Depressive Disorders. In Holland J, Breitbart
WS, Butow PN, et al., eds. *Psycho-Oncology*. New York: Oxford University
Press, 2015:280–287.

Gelenberg AJ. Using assessment tools to screen for, diagnose, and treat
major depressive disorder in clinical practice. *J Clin Psychiatry* 2010; 71[Suppl
E1]:e01.

Robinson S, Kissane D, Brooker J, Burney S. A systematic review of the demoral-
ization syndrome in individuals with progressive disease and cancer: a decade
of research. *J Pain Symptom Management* 2014; 49(3):595–610.

Diarrhea and Anorectal Problems

**SITUATION: Frequent watery or excessively loose stools,
anorectal irritation, pain, or pruritus**

Causes

- Overtreatment of constipation or adverse effect of laxative regimen
- Fecal impaction (overflow incontinence)
- Related to diet/enteral feeding
- Related to drugs, including antibiotic-associated diarrhea
- Infectious (viral, fungal, bacterial, including *Clostridium difficile*)
- Partial bowel obstruction
- Related to specific tumor (pancreatic neuroendocrine, carcinoid,
  pheochromocytoma)
- Post-gastrectomy "dumping" syndrome
- Pancreatic insufficiency
- Malabsorption related to surgical procedures (colectomy, ileal resection,
  gastric bypass)
- Post-radiation or chemotherapy syndrome
- Anorectal tumors
- GI bleeding
- Post–celiac plexus block
- HIV-related noninfectious diarrhea

Findings

- Frequent liquid stool (more than three or four bowel movements in 24 hours)
- Abdominal cramping
- Hyperactive bowel sounds
- Anal pain, burning, irritation, itching, tenesmus (feeling of incomplete evacuation)
- Anal lesions/hemorrhoids/fissures

Assessment

Biomedical

- Determine usual bowel habits and patterns, extent of change, and duration of symptoms.
- Review bowel regimen (cathartics, laxatives, stool softeners).
- Review current medications (metoclopramide, SSRIs, antibiotics, antacids, proton pump inhibitors, thyroid hormone).
- Review dietary intake and past history of bowel disorders, including celiac disease, inflammatory and irritable bowel disease.
- Consider testing to rule out hyperthyroidism or signs of or history of thyroid disease, or if patient is on thyroid medication.
- Determine relationship between current disease process and propensity for bowel dysfunction.
- Systems review for concomitant fever/nausea/vomiting/abdominal pain, blood in stool, number of bowel movements, consistency/color/odor/quality of stool (floating or greasy stool, clay-like, etc.)
- Auscultate bowel sounds and gently palpate abdomen for abnormal findings.
- Visually examine perineum and anus, and perform digital examination to determine presence of fecal impaction.
- General examination to determine if patient is dehydrated: tongue and mucous membranes, skin turgor, orthostatic blood pressure/pulse changes

Psychosocial

- Assess for patient anxiety and distress over need for personal care due to diarrhea and anorectal conditions.
- Assess for feelings of shame/embarrassment due to fecal incontinence.

Processes of Care

Practical and Biomedical

- General
  a. Notify physician if new or rapidly advancing signs/symptoms (e.g., abdominal distention, suspected bowel obstruction, GI bleeding, severe dehydration, etc.)
  b. Discontinue cathartics/laxatives/prokinetics (metoclopramide) as well as other medications that may be contributing until symptoms abate, and then reinstitute gradually.

   c. Assess for enteral feeding as a cause for diarrhea.

   d. Clear fluids with slowly advancing diet as symptoms allow and appetite dictates. Avoid dairy products, spicy foods, fatty foods, caffeine, and alcohol.

   d. Rehydrate orally with oral hydration solution, clear liquids, sports drinks, broth.

   e. Consider subcutaneous infusion (hypodermoclysis) if prognosis warrants:

     1. Normal saline infused at 0.5 to 1.0 ml/kg/hr with a maximum rate of 60 ml/hr, using a 25-gauge butterfly needle inserted at a 45-degree angle to the skin, or a subcutaneous "button" device. Can add hyaluronidase 500 units/L if readily available to enhance absorption (although randomized studies have not shown significant benefit of its use).

   f. Consider IV fluids if patient has IV access.

- Nonspecific pharmacotherapy

   a. Kaopectate 30 ml every 30 to 60 minutes until diarrhea stops; maximum eight doses/day

   b. Loperamide HCl (Imodium AD) 1 tablet = 2 mg, 5 ml liquid = 1 mg. 4 mg PO initially, then 2 mg PO after each loose stool. Maximum 16 tablets/24 hours.

   c. Diphenoxylate HCl 2.5 mg/atropine 0.025 mg (Lomotil) one or two tablets or 5 to 10 ml PO up to four times daily. Maintenance 2 tablets or 10 ml daily.

   d. Add fiber supplement to increase bulk to stool (if no risk of bowel obstruction) such as psyllium (Metamucil) or methylcellulose (Citrocel).

   e. For intractable diarrhea: Octreotide 100 to 300 mcg SQ tid or q24hr by continuous infusion; maximum 1,500 mcg/24 hours

   f. Probiotics

    — May reduce severity of diarrhea in patients with advanced disease but could be a rare cause of sepsis in cancer patients; further evidence is needed to recommend them

    — May help reduce diarrhea in patients on enteral feeding

- Etiology-specific approaches to therapy

   a. Carcinoid and other neuroendocrine tumors

    — Octreotide is the mainstay of treatment: 100 to 300 mcg SQ tid or 300 to 900 mcg q24hr by continuous infusion, titrate slowly; maximum 1,500 mcg/24 hours

   b. Short bowel syndrome

    — Cholestyramine may decrease diarrhea if patient has had a distal ileal resection with bile acid diarrhea.

    — Octreotide for refractory diarrhea

   c. Dumping syndrome (post-gastrectomy)

    — Small, low-carbohydrate meals; avoid simple carbohydrates (sugar, sweets, soda, candy, sports drink)

    — Dietary fiber supplementation or 5 g of pectin with each meal

    — Restrict fluid intake during meals and for at least 30 minutes after meals.

    — Octreotide for refractory diarrhea

d. Pancreatic insufficiency (post–Whipple procedure or total pancreatectomy)
   — Low-fat diet
   — Pancreatic enzyme replacement: generally 10,000 to 30,000 IU of pancreatic lipase with meals
e. Post-radiation or chemotherapy syndrome
   — Eliminate fiber and dairy products.
   — NSAIDs (e.g., ibuprofen, celecoxib) to counteract inflammatory effects leading to radiation enteritis if tolerated and not contraindicated
   — Progressive trial of loperamide, diphenoxylate/atropine, octreotide for diarrhea, titrated to control symptoms
   — Ganglion impar block has been reported to be successful for severe anorectal pain due to radiation proctitis.
f. Antibiotic-associated diarrhea caused by *C. difficile*
   — Discontinue unnecessary antibiotics.
   — For mild to moderate disease: metronidazole 500 mg PO tid for 10 to 14 days
   — For severe disease: vancomycin 125 mg PO qid for 10 to 14 days
   — For severe complicated disease: vancomycin 500 mg PO qid plus metronidazole 500 mg IV q8hr
   — Contact precautions (gowns and gloves) and careful handwashing with soap and water (alcohol-based sanitizing solution is not adequate)
g. Candidiasis of the anogenital region (due to immunosuppression or antibiotic therapy)
   — Miconazole or clotrimazole cream topically tid or fluconazole 150 mg PO daily for 3 days
h. Anal irritation/hemorrhoids/fissures
   — Warm water, nonabrasive cleansing and thorough drying
   — Apply zinc oxide or A&D ointment to unbroken skin.
   — Apply corticosteroid cream, foam, or suppositories (preparations with or without local anesthetic) to macerated or inflamed skin or to rectal hemorrhoids for up to 3 days.
   — For severe pruritus ani, use a sedating antihistamine such as promethazine 12.5 mg PO q HS or doxepin 10 to 25 mg PO q HS.
   — Topical nitroglycerin cream 0.2% to 0.4% for anal fissures: available as Rectiv (0.4% nitroglycerin) ointment or by diluting 2% ointment with petroleum jelly (possible side effect is headache)
i. Rectal tumors
   — If prognosis warrants, consider palliative radiation therapy or endoscopic laser therapy.
   — Hydrocortisone foam, one applicator PR bid
   — EMLA cream or other topical local anesthetic formulation prn

Goals/Outcomes

- Regular well-formed stools to the extent possible, limited only by underlying disease and patient tolerance/preference of interventions
- Ability to ingest foods of choice without undue discomfort or diarrhea
- Absence of perineal/anal discomfort

Documentation in the Medical Record

Initial Assessment

- Number and character of bowel movements
- Likely etiology of diarrhea
- Contributing factors to diarrhea
- Other anorectal symptoms (pain, irritation, itching)
- Medication review
- Patient/caregiver approaches to controlling diarrhea
- Findings from physical examination

Interdisciplinary Progress Notes

- Therapies applied and results of interventions
- Findings from reassessment: frequency/quality of bowel movements and associated symptoms; physical examination

IDT Care Plan

- Interventions planned and schedule of reassessments
- Contingency plans

Recommended Reading

Abernethy A. Management of gastrointestinal symptoms in advanced cancer patients: the rapid learning cancer clinical model. *Curr Opin Support Palliat Care* 2010; 4(1):36–45.

Blazer A. Diarrhoea in the critically ill. *Curr Opin Critical Care* 2015; 21(2):142–153.

Bowen P. Using subcutaneous fluids in end-of-life care. *Nursing Times* 2014; 110(40):12–14.

Jain V. Gastrointestinal side effects of prescription medications in the older adult. *J Clin Gastroenterol* 2009; 43(2):103–110.

Khosla A. Successful treatment of radiation-induced proctitis pain by blockade of the ganglion impar in an elderly patient with prostate cancer: a case report. *Pain Med* 2013; 14(5):662–666.

Prommer E. Established and potential therapeutic applications of octreotide in palliative care. *Support Care Cancer* 2008; 16:1117–1123.

Redman MG. The efficacy and safety of probiotics in people with cancer, a systematic review. *Ann Oncol* 2014; 25:1919–1929.

Shaw C, Taylor L. Treatment-related diarrhea in patients with cancer. *Clin J Oncol Nurs* 2012; 16(4):413–417.

Von Guten CF, Gafford E. Treatment of non-pain-related symptoms. *Cancer J* 2013; 19(5):397–404.

Whelan K. Mechanisms, prevention, and management of diarrhea in enteral nutrition. *Curr Opin Gastroenterol* 2011; 27:152–159.

Dysphagia and Oropharyngeal Problems

SITUATION: Choking with eating or drinking, difficult or painful swallowing, mucositis, oral candidiasis (thrush), and other painful

or distressing/disturbing oropharyngeal conditions associated
with advanced disease

Causes

- Dysphagia, with or without oral candidiasis or mucositis, commonly occurs in:
  a. Patients with cancers of the head and neck or the GI tract, and those involving mediastinal structures
  b. Patients who have undergone radiation treatments to the head and neck, the GI tract, or mediastinal structures
  c. Patients with surgical changes to the head, neck, or thoracic structures
  d. Patients who are severely immunocompromised (e.g., AIDS, post-chemotherapy, steroid therapy)
  e. Patients who have progressive neuromuscular diseases (e.g., amyotrophic lateral sclerosis [ALS])
  f. Patients who have cerebrovascular disease (post-stroke)
  g. Patients with structural anatomy problems, including Zenker's diverticulum or achalasia
  h. Patients with poor dentition and oral hygiene
  i. Patients experiencing medication-induced dystonic reactions
  j. Patients subjected to polypharmacy, especially with medications causing sedation, muscle relaxation, or xerostomia
  k. Patients with respiratory compromise or who have recently been extubated
  l. Patients with a history of severe reflux, heartburn, or repeated pneumonia

Findings

- Excessive secretions, drooling
- Falling asleep during meals
- Holding food in the mouth, or excessive duration of chewing
- Painful and/or uncoordinated swallowing
- Avoidance of food or beverages
- Choking, coughing, excessive throat clearing during meals
- Increased respiratory rate or labored breathing during meals
- Increased congestion after meals
- Food pocketed in the cheeks or under the tongue
- Panting or other postures indicating difficulty in managing oral secretions and swallowing
- Whitish patches (plaques) in oral cavity (tongue, mucosal surface, gingiva) that scrape off and have a beefy red base
- Erythematous oral mucosa without plaques (atrophic candidiasis)
- Taste perversion

Assessment

- History and systems review pertinent to upper GI system, including sense of taste, quality and intensity of pain, difficulties with chewing and swallowing
- History of pneumonia
- History of previous swallowing problems and dietary modifications

- History of changes in vocal pitch or new vocal breathiness (may indicate new vocal-fold dysfunction)
- Examination of oropharynx: observe for signs of candida, other lesions, fit of dentures, odor (halitosis), posterior pharyngeal erythema indicating possible irritation from reflux, or pocketed food from an earlier meal
- Observe patient manage own secretions during history taking, and observe patient during the act of swallowing.
- Observe bedding for evidence of residue from previous meals or pills on the pillowcase or sheets.
- Review medications for possible dystonic reactions from phenothiazines, butyrophenones, etc. (e.g., prochlorperazine, chlorpromazine, haloperidol, droperidol).
- Review medications for muscle relaxants, anticholinergics, diuretics, hypnotics, sedatives and their timing as related to meals.

Processes of Care

Practical

- Optimize positioning for drinking and eating (sitting if possible, or elevated head of bed).
  - Allow the patient a short rest after positioning before food is offered.
  - Place food in the unaffected side of the mouth if applicable.
- Frequent small sips during meals; crushed ice; refresh bedside beverages/ice frequently
- Alternate bites and sips to clear food from posterior pharynx.
- Use care with or avoid straws if the patient tends to gulp liquids.
- Frequent rest breaks during meals
- Mouth care after each meal
- Have patient avoid excessively sour (acidic) or hot fluids/meals until symptoms remit. Soft, cool meals (yogurt, cottage cheese, pudding, ice cream) may be all that is tolerated.
- Evaluate for need to thicken liquids; commercially available starch-based or gum-containing thickeners are available to thicken liquids.
- Avoid mixed-consistency foods like stew as these take considerable coordination to chew and swallow the consistency mix (both solid and liquid components in a single bite).
- Consider Speech Pathology consult to customize dietary consistency modifications, to develop compensatory postures/strategies to maximize eating safety, to retrain swallowing to the extent possible, and to train caregivers in safety techniques.
- Dietary/nutritionist consultation to maximize nutrition within parameters of the dysphagia

Biomedical

- For dystonia, if symptom-causing medication is still indicated, initiate therapy with diphenhydramine 25 to 50 mg PO/IV qid or benztropine 1 to 2 mg PO/IV qd or bid.

- For painful oral candidiasis and mucositis, use opioid analgesics as needed to control pain until antifungal therapy has been effective; a 1:2:8 mixture of diphenhydramine elixir/lidocaine (2% to 4%)/Maalox as a swish-and-swallow suspension provides temporary relief of symptoms and might lessen the need for opioid analgesics, especially prior to mealtimes.
- Edema, inflammation, tumor burden: consider corticosteroids and H_2 blockers (potential benefit of corticosteroids must be balanced against associated risks of immunosuppression)
- For candidiasis
  1. Topical treatment with clotrimazole 10-mg troches, 5 doses/day, can be initiated as symptoms and patient compliance allow.
  2. If symptoms do not rapidly abate or patient compliance does not allow topical antifungal therapy, fluconazole 150 mg PO followed by 100 mg PO daily for 5 days
- For intractable oral bleeding: if available, apply topical thrombin to hemorrhagic areas; consider tranexamic acid 500 to 1,000 mg PO tid or aminocaproic acid 5 g PO followed by 1 g PO qid (see "Bleeding, Oozing, and Malodorous Lesions" earlier in this section)
- Severe halitosis should be treated to prevent reluctance to provide care, social isolation, humiliation, and nausea:
  1. Frequent prophylactic care (cleansing of dentures and oropharynx)
  2. Antimicrobial mouthwash or half-strength hydrogen peroxide gargle
  3. Metronidazole 250 to 500 mg PO tid or applied as a topical gel (0.75%), if feasible, to putrid necrotic or fungating lesions for control of anaerobic colonization (see "Bleeding, Draining, and Malodorous Lesions" earlier in this section)
  4. Broad-spectrum antibiotics (e.g., trimethoprim-sulfa; cephalosporin) for foul-smelling, purulent bronchopulmonary sputum/secretions
  5. Treat reflux.
  6. Elevate the head of the bed with low blocks if needed for reflux control.

Goals/Outcomes

- Decrease pain, hunger, and fear/struggles at mealtimes
- Normalize swallowing and control of secretions as much as disease status allows
- Reduce likelihood of an aspiration event to the extent disease allows
- Improve enjoyment of food and beverages
- Improve ability to talk
- Reduce social isolation, embarrassment, nausea

Documentation in the Medical Record

Initial Assessment

- History of difficulty with swallowing or managing secretions, choking
- Type and quantity of food/beverage intake causing both most problems and also best success
- Time of day problems exist (e.g., worse as the day progresses) if applicable
- Pain in mouth, throat, or mediastinum

Physical Examination Findings

- Patient/caregiver ability to cope with symptoms/interventions
- Patient ability to ingest oral or buccal medications; possible need for liquid forms of pills/capsules and/or transdermal, SQ, or IV dosage forms

Interdisciplinary Progress Notes

- Interventions recommended and tried and outcomes
- Results of evaluations and caregiver observations
- Patient/caregiver difficulties with compliance
- Findings from repeat physical examinations

IDT Care Plan

- Specific interventions for each identified symptom
- Oral hygiene plan
- Contingency plans
- Planned modifications to any religious, spiritual, or other rituals needed because of the dysphagia/odynophagia
- Schedule of follow-up visits/examinations

Recommended Reading

Altman KW. Understanding dysphagia: a rapidly emerging problem. *Otolaryngol Clin North Am* 2013; 46(6):xiii–xvi.

Giles M, Barker M, Hayes A. The role of the speech-language pathologist in home care. *Home Healthcare Nurse* 2014; 32(6):349–353.

Liantonio J, Salzman B, Snyderman D. Preventing aspiration by addressing three key risk factors: dysphagia, poor oral hygiene, and medication use. *Ann Long Term Care Clin Care Aging* 2014; 22(10) 42–48.

Rudakiewicz J. Methods for managing residents with dysphagia. *Nursing Older People* 2015; 27(4):29–33.

Vallons KJ, Helmens HJ, Oudhuis AA. Effect of human saliva on the consistency of thickened drinks for individuals with dysphagia. *Int J Lang Commun Disord* 2015; 50(2):165–175.

Edema: Peripheral Edema, Ascites, and Lymphedema

SITUATION: Peripheral edema, ascites, or lymphedema that results in physical or emotional distress or functional impairment or adds difficulty to caregiving

Causes

- Ascites and lymphedema
  - Primary neoplasm (ovary, breast, endometrium, colon, stomach, pancreas, bronchus, hepatobiliary)
  - Right heart failure

- Metastasis to peritoneum or liver
- Venous or lymphatic obstruction/occlusion due to neoplasm
- Portal hypertension secondary to advanced liver disease
- Chylous ascites (lymph plus emulsified fat and white blood cells) from lymphatic obstruction or abdominal lymphoma
- Postsurgical or radiotherapy-induced lymphatic obstruction
- Peripheral edema
  - Hypoalbuminemia
  - Chronic steroid therapy
  - Renal failure
  - Congestive heart failure
  - Circulatory impairment from inadequate mobility/prolonged dependency
  - Fluid overload from artificial nutrition
  - Chronic peripheral vascular disease/post-thrombosis syndrome
  - Cor pulmonale (right heart failure) due to advanced pulmonary disease
  - Acute phlebitis
  - Thyroid disease
  - Drug induced (e.g., nonsteroidal anti-inflammatories [NSAIDs], cortico-steroids, cyclosporine)

Findings

- Ascites
  - Feelings of bloating, regurgitation, or reflux
  - Early satiety and nausea
  - Increased abdominal girth, shifting dullness, fluid wave, caput medusae (engorged venous plexus visible on abdominal wall in severe cases of portal hypertension)
  - Lower extremity/genital swelling
  - Orthopnea and dyspnea as ascites progresses
- Lymphedema or peripheral edema
  - Swelling of distal extremities with pitting of skin when gentle pressure is applied
  - Presence of fluid accumulation in dependent body parts (e.g., presacral area in bed-bound patients)
  - Unilateral extremity swelling in postsurgical or post-radiotherapy lymphedema
  - Tight and shiny skin with visible fluid extrusion in severe cases
  - Jugular venous distention
  - Pain with acute phlebitis
  - Electrolyte abnormalities

Assessment

- Assess cardiovascular status (e.g., vital signs, cardiac rate, rhythm, mur-murs, rubs, gallops, jugular veins, peripheral pulses, peripheral perfusion).
- Examine dependent body parts and extremities.
- Auscultate lungs for rales, rubs, and decreased breath sounds.
- Examine abdomen for findings of ascites.

- Assess fluid balance (volume in, urine out), when appropriate; consider benefit versus burden of serum electrolyte and protein assessment.
- Assess weight changes, when feasible.
- Assess for tachypnea and respiratory distress.
- Evaluate for symptoms of reflux.
- Determine association between body position and physical signs and symptoms of distress.

Processes of Care

Practical and Biomedical

- Ascites
- Pharmacotherapy: worth a trial, but effects may be marginal, especially in malignant ascites
  1. Diuretics
     a. Spironolactone 100 mg PO daily up to 200 mg bid. If needed, add:
     b. Furosemide 40 to 240 mg PO daily; continuous infusion of 100 mg/ 24 hr IV is an alternative; balance benefits against potential adverse effects, such as volume depletion and electrolyte disturbance
        - Patients with soft edema who have failed to respond to medical management with diuretics can be treated with subcutaneous needle drainage.
        - Symptomatic ascites that is intractable to diuretic therapy and subcutaneous needle drainage may require large-volume paracentesis at the bedside, but relief is usually temporary, so consider an intraperitoneal catheter if appropriate.
- If highly symptomatic ascites reaccumulates quickly and the patient is not imminently dying, discuss regarding the placement of a semipermanent catheter for continuous drainage, acknowledging the burdens associated with such a procedure (transport to a day-surgery facility; discomfort from the operative procedure; risk of infection, occlusion, and dislodgment).
- Peritoneo-venous shunting (PVS) may have a place in malignant ascites. The cytologic status of ascites should be considered in selection for PVS, as a shunt half-life is significantly greater in cytologically negative ascites; contraindications include loculated ascites, jaundice, infection, hemorrhagic ascites or ascitic fluid protein greater than 50 g/L, pseudomyxoma peritonei, and coagulopathy.
- Lymphedema: Primary treatment consists of nonpharmacological approaches:
  - Postural support
  - Maintaining range of motion with active or passive physical therapy, if tolerated
  - Compression bandaging/gloves/stockings/pneumatic devices,
  - Manual lymphatic drainage
- Peripheral edema
  - Review current diuretic and cardiac medications with physician, and adjust appropriately (see earlier).
  - Elevate legs prn unless contraindicated by compromised cardiac function.

- Turn and reposition recumbent patients q2hr as tolerated.
- Consider relative benefits/burdens of decreasing fluid intake.
- Consider need for daily potassium supplement when patient is on long-term diuretic therapy.
- Consider antibiotic therapy if cellulitis is present.
- Notify physician if findings of acute thrombophlebitis are present.
- Some end-stage kidney failure patients who choose not to start dialysis, or decide to discontinue it, may benefit from maximizing furosemide diuretics and adding metolazone 2.5 to 5 mg/day.
- In refractory situations in which the symptom burden justifies a more aggressive approach and the patient wishes to pursue such an approach, stenting the superior vena cava can, in some cases, relieve associated upper-extremity edema. In the case of malignant ascites, an intraperitoneal catheter/gastrostomy/peritoneal port may help terminal patients with symptom relief. These procedures may be required unexpectedly and urgently, and so, as with other highly specialized procedures, it is advisable to establish these types of consultancy contacts and relationships in advance of actually needing them.

Goals/Outcomes

- Reduce ascites, lymphedema, and peripheral edema to the greatest extent with the least invasive approaches possible in order to minimize physical and emotional distress, improve patient physical functioning, and facilitate caregiving

Documentation in the Medical Record

Initial Assessment

- Results of systems review and physical examination
- Intensity and types of physical and emotional distress, functional loss to patient imposed by ascites/lymphedema/peripheral edema
- Degree of burden imposed by untreated signs/symptoms on caregiver

Interdisciplinary Progress Notes

- Content of discussion regarding treatment options
- Types and results of interventions

IDT Care Plan

- Defined goals of therapies
- Specific interventions and contingency plans

Recommended Reading

Bar-Sela G, Omer A, Flechter E, et al. Treatment of lower extremity edema by subcutaneous drainage in palliative care of advanced cancer patients. *Am J Hosp Palliat Care* 2010; 27(4):272–275.

Beck M, Wanchai A, Stewart BR, et al. Palliative care for cancer-related lymphedema: a systematic review. *J Palliat Med* 2012; 15(7):821–827.

Beng TS, Chin LE. Multiple subcutaneous puncture and stoma bag drainage for gross lower limb edema: A case report. *J Palliat Med* 2010; 13(8):1037–1038.

Cheng HW, Sham MK. Case series: combination therapy with low dose metolazone and furosemide. *Int Urol Nephrol* 2014; 46(9):1809–1813.

Coupe NA, Cox K, Clark K, et al. Outcomes of permanent peritoneal ports for the management of recurrent malignant ascites. *J Palliat Med* 2013; 16(8):938–940.

Duvnjak S, Andersen P. Endovascular treatment of superior vena cava syndrome. *Int Angiol* 2011; 30(5):458–610.

O'Connor OJ, Driver E, McDermott S, et al. Palliative gastrostomy in the setting of voluminous ascites. *J Palliat Med* 2014; 17(7):811–821.

Shaw C, Bassett RL, Fox PS, et al. Palliative venting gastrostomy in patients with malignant bowel obstruction and ascites. *Ann Surg Oncol* 2013; 20(2):497–505.

Fatigue, Weakness (Aesthenia), and Excessive Sedation

SITUATION: The patient's quality of life is severely affected by fatigue, weakness, or diminished energy due to advancing disease.

Causes

- Most chronic disease states in the far-advanced stages (e.g., cancer, COPD, heart failure, renal failure, hepatic failure) lead to a state of aesthenia, characterized by chronic fatigue and weakness; these continue to be some of the most challenging symptoms to manage effectively, once pain is under control.
- Catabolic nutritional state due to disease factors
- Hypoxemia or inadequate oxygen-carrying capacity (decreased red cell mass)
- Clinical depression should be ruled out since the symptoms of depression may mimic aesthenia (see "Depression" earlier in this section).
- Medications: Anticholinergics, antihistamines, benzodiazepines and other sleep aids, and neuroleptics commonly cause fatigue and sedation; antihypertensive therapy that may have been appropriate previously may cause excessive reduction in blood pressure in debilitated patients with weight loss, resulting in marked fatigue and postural hypotension.
- Excessive use of alcohol may go unrecognized, especially in the elderly, or may be viewed as benign in chronically ill patients.
- Boredom: Absence of stimulation is very common in homebound and especially bedridden patients, and can mimic depression.

Findings

- Weakness, lethargy, fatigue, hypersomnolence after minimal or no activity

Assessment

Biomedical

- Simple measures should be used to find and treat reversible or easily treatable causes of severe fatigue, lethargy, and weakness (e.g., metabolic disturbances, anemia, hypoxemia) when the context is appropriate (i.e., life expectancy will allow meaningful benefit from testing and therapeutic intervention). In patients with rapid decline from life-limiting diseases, the luxury of an exhaustive evaluation is not always feasible or in the patient's best interest. In these cases, or where reversible processes are not present or specifically directed therapies are not possible, empiric therapy is indicated.

- Review current medications and determine if there are any changes that, on balance, might lead to overall benefits.
- Evaluate muscle tone and strength; unless myopathic weakness is the result of ongoing corticosteroid therapy, this class of drugs can palliate symptoms of weakness and fatigue for a short time (days to weeks).

Psychosocial/Spiritual

- Determine patient/caregiver perceptions and level of distress imposed by degree of fatigue and weakness.
- Determine to what degree important short-term goals are being impeded by symptoms.

Processes of Care

Biomedical

- Consider and discuss benefits and burdens of red cell transfusion if anemia is a likely contributing cause of symptoms.
- Use supplemental oxygen only if a therapeutic trial proves beneficial when hypoxemia is determined to be the cause of symptoms.
- In patients with heart failure, review medical management and determine if there are any adjustments in cardiotropic drugs that may improve end-organ perfusion, balancing benefits/burdens and patient preferences.
- Palliative pharmacotherapy
  - **Psychostimulants**: The psychostimulant methylphenidate has been shown to be beneficial in open trials, with inconclusive results in placebo-controlled trials. It may be especially useful in balancing therapeutic analgesic effects of opioids against excessive daytime sedation, allowing upward dose titration of opioids as needed for pain control. Other stimulants (e.g., dexamphetamine, modafinil) have been reported by clinicians to be beneficial, but the literature does not provide high-quality evidence for efficacy. If these agents are determined to be potentially useful, then close follow-up and monitoring for incipient signs of psychosis, agitation, or sleep disturbance are obligatory when initiating and titrating such therapy.
    - Methylphenidate 2.5 mg PO every morning to start, or
    - Dextroamphetamine 2.5 mg PO every morning to start, or
    - Modafinil 200 mg PO every morning
  - **Corticosteroids**: Dexamethasone and methylprednisolone have been evaluated and found to have a positive effect on fatigue, appetite, and patient satisfaction.
  - **Additional agents**: Other agents that have some anecdotal clinical evidence supporting potential reduction of chronic disease–related fatigue include acetylsalicylic acid, amantadine, L-carnitine.

Psychosocial/Spiritual

- Provide realistic information about the natural history of the disease process being experienced, with aesthenia being a usual and expected consequence.
- Help organize patient/caregiver routines to conserve energy and pace activities. Address the potential value of hiring aides.
- Review the role of energy-sparing devices such as a walker, wheelchair, or motorized scooter; patients may be reluctant to use such devices because they visibly represent loss of functional capacity, so this may be an ongoing discussion and reorientation of values in order to preserve dignity.
- Help set limits on social visits if they seem to be more exhausting than helpful.
- Help reset goals to a level that is more attainable based on the patient's capabilities.
- Consider occupational therapy evaluation to determine if there is any form of stimulation that might be beneficial; use volunteers to carry on such a program to counteract boredom.
- Formal rehabilitation programs may improve function in patients with cancer and cardiopulmonary disease and may be appropriate for patients with a more extended prognosis; in fact, physical exercise, yoga, and dance have all been demonstrated to have a positive effect on fatigue in the palliative care setting.

Goals/Outcomes

- Maximize patient energy based on the course of disease, in keeping with patient preferences
- Decreased frustration with clinical circumstances beyond patient/caregiver/professional control
- Patient feels free from having to perform at an unrealistic level of expectation
- Identify short-term goals (whatever they are—even simply "being") that are attainable and lead the patient to feel that his/her existence has value

Documentation in the Medical Record

Initial Assessment

- Description of patient's level of fatigue, functional capabilities
- Determination if goals and expectations are realistic
- Degree of acceptance versus frustration with clinical circumstances
- Identification of factors contributing to fatigue, weakness (pacing, length of social visits, structure and schedule of activities throughout the day)

Interdisciplinary Progress Notes

- Content of discussions, ongoing evaluations, interventions
- Results of interventions

IDT Care Plan

- Specific interventions and role of IDT members in helping to manage coping issues

Recommended Reading

Mucke M, Mochamat, Cuhls H, et al. Pharmacological treatments for fatigue associated with palliative care. *Cochrane Collaboration*, Wiley and Sons, LTD, May 30, 2015.

Oldervoll LM, Loge JH, Lydersen S, et al. Physical exercise for cancer patients with advanced disease: a randomized controlled trial. *Oncologist* 2011; 16:1649.

Paulsen O, Klepstad P, Rosland JH, et al. Efficacy of methylprednisolone on pain, fatigue, and appetite loss in patients with advanced cancer using opioids: a randomized, placebo-controlled, double-blind trial. *J Clin Oncol* 2014; 32(29):3221.

Selman LE, Williams J, Simms V. A mixed-methods evaluation of complementary therapy services in palliative care: yoga and dance therapy. *Eur J Cancer Care (Engl)* 2012; 21:87.

Shaygannejad V, Janghorbani M, Ashtari F, Zakeri H. Comparison of the effect of aspirin and amantadine for the treatment of fatigue in multiple sclerosis: a randomized, blinded, crossover study. *Neurol Res* 2012; 34(9):854–858.

Yennurajalingam S, Frisbee-Hume S, Delgado-Guay MO, et al. Dexamethasone (DM) for cancer-related fatigue: A double-blinded, randomized, placebo-controlled trial. *J Clin Oncol* 2013; 31(25):3076–3082.

Yennurajalingam S, Kang JH, Cheng HY, et al. Characteristics of advanced cancer patients with cancer-related fatigue enrolled in clinical trials and patients referred to outpatient palliative care clinics. *J Pain Symptom Manage* 2013; 45(3):534–541.

Fever, Flushing, and Diaphoresis

SITUATION: Fever, flushing, and/or diaphoresis associated with terminal illness

Fever is an elevation of body temperature due to normal thermoregulatory mechanisms. The hypothalamus regulates heat production and dissipation to keep body temperature within a specific range. Cytokines, which are produced in response to infection, inflammation, injury, or immune reactions, cause the hypothalamus to raise the normal body temperature to febrile levels. Chills and sweating accompany fever, but sweating can occur independently of fever. Elevated body temperature can also occur due to failure of normal thermoregulation; this is referred to as hyperpyrexia. Hot flashes are episodic, sudden sensations of heat, intense sweating, and flushing and are commonly associated with menopause.

Causes

- Infection
  - Viral: upper respiratory, pneumonia, HIV, hepatitis C
  - Bacterial: urinary tract, pneumonia, cellulitis, sepsis, abscess (often intraabdominal). Less common: osteomyelitis, endocarditis.
  - Mycobacterial: tuberculosis, atypical mycobacterial
  - Fungal
- Malignancy: tumor-related fever or night sweats from release of pro-inflammatory cytokines such as TNF and interleukins (IL-1, IL-6)
  - Lymphoma
  - Leukemia

- Solid tumors: many, but most common are renal cell carcinoma, germ cell, medullary thyroid, and neuroendocrine tumors
  - Liver metastasis
- Hot flashes due to estrogen or androgen deficiency
  - Breast cancer after oophorectomy
  - Prostate cancer after orchiectomy or androgen-depletion therapies
- Medications
  - Drug-induced hypersensitivity reactions: Hypersensitivity is the most common cause of drug fever, and almost any drug can cause fever due to hypersensitivity. Common medications causing drug fever are anticonvulsants, antimicrobial (beta-lactams, sulfonamides, and nitrofurantoin), and allopurinol.
  - Drug-induced sweating: opioids, antidepressants (SSRIs, SNRIs, tricyclics), insulin, theophylline, omeprazole, calcium channel blockers, hydralazine, donepezil, levodopa
- Hyperpyrexia due to drug toxicities causing altered thermoregulation
  - Serotonin syndrome: associated with SSRIs, tramadol, ondansetron, metoclopramide, tryptans, dextromethorphan, cyclobenzaprine, fentanyl. Symptoms include hyperthermia, agitation, diaphoresis, tremors, hyperreflexia.
  - Neuroleptic malignant syndrome: associated with typical and atypical antipsychotics, phenothiazine antiemetics. Symptoms include hyperthermia, altered mental status, muscle rigidity, diaphoresis.
  - Anticholinergic toxicity: associated with antihistamines, tricyclic antidepressants, oxybutynin, tolterodine, scopolamine, glycopyrrolate, promethazine, chlorpromazine. Symptoms include hyperpyrexia, delirium, urinary retention, tachycardia. In contrast to serotonin syndrome and neuroleptic malignant syndrome, there is no sweating.
- Substance withdrawal causing sweating
  - Opioid withdrawal
  - Alcohol withdrawal
  - Benzodiazepine withdrawal
  - Cocaine withdrawal
- Endocrine disorders
  - Hyperthyroidism
  - Hypoglycemia
  - Menopause
- Neurologic disorders
  - Stroke
  - Autonomic neuropathy
- Miscellaneous
  - Temporal arteritis
  - Autoimmune conditions

Findings

- Elevated body temperature—normal body temperature ranges within 1 degree of 37°C and has diurnal variation. A temperature greater than 38°C (100.4°F) is considered a fever. A fever greater than 38.3°C (101°F) for greater than 3 weeks is considered a "fever of unknown origin."

- Headache, muscle/joint pain, dizziness
- Tachycardia
- Altered mental status (decreased level of consciousness or agitation/rest-lessness, fitful sleep)
- Diaphoresis (sweating) with or without fever
- Flushing, warm skin
- Hot flashes: episodic flushing and sweating

Assessment

- Systems review and physical examination to rule out infection (e.g., urinary tract, respiratory tract, cellulitis, intraabdominal abscess, osteomyelitis)
- Specific disease states that may be cause of fever/diaphoresis—malignancy, neurologic, endocrine, autoimmune
- Review of medications as potential cause of fever/diaphoresis/hyperpyrexia

Processes of Care

Practical

- Increase room air circulation and give cool sponge baths.
- Cool wet towels (avoid ice packs due to discomfort)
- Remove heavy bedclothes and bedding.
- Provide mouth care: use toothette dipped in fluid of choice to moisten mouth and apply lip balm to keep lips from cracking.

Biomedical

- Antibiotic therapy if obvious source of infection is suspected based on goals of care
- Pharmacotherapeutic approaches
    1. Antipyretics
        a. Acetaminophen 650 mg PO/PR q4–6hr around the clock. Body weight less than 50 kg: 15 mg/kg q6hr or 12.5 mg/kg q4hr. Maximum 3,000 mg/day (according to current U.S. FDA guidance). Use with caution in hepatic impairment.
        b. NSAIDs: Ibuprofen, naproxen, and indomethacin are equally effective for tumor-related fever; however, naproxen sodium has the most rapid effect. Dosage: Ibuprofen 10 mg/kg PO q6–8hr; maximum daily dose 40 mg/kg. Naproxen sodium 220 to 440 mg q8–12hr; do not exceed 15 mg/kg/day. Indomethacin 25 to 75 mg/dose PO or PR two or three times daily (rectal suppositories are 50 mg); maximum dose 200 mg daily. Use NSAIDs with caution in renal, hepatic, and cardiac disease.
    2. Treatment of rigors (shaking chills) is empiric. Some suggested approaches:
        a. Meperidine 0.25 to 0.5 mg/kg IV/IM/SQ prn *(NOTE: this is an exception to the usual injunction against the use of meperidine)*
        b. Promethazine 12.5 to 25 mg PO/IM/IV or 25 to 50 mg PR q6–8hr prn

3. For suspected tumor- or metastasis-induced diaphoresis (e.g., liver metastasis)
   a. NSAIDs (see dosages above)
   b. Steroid: dexamethasone 2 to 4 mg once or twice a day, prednisone 5 to 20 mg once or twice a day
   c. Thioridazine 10 to 25 mg q HS
   d. Gabapentin 600 to 1,800 mg (usual dose 300 mg tid)
4. For opioid-related sweating (based on case reports in the literature)
   a. Opioid rotation is not effective.
   b. Desloratidine 5 mg daily
   c. Scopolamine patch q72hr
   d. Olanzapine 5 mg bid
5. For sweating due to SSRIs/SNRIs
   a. Change to a different SSRI or SNRI or to mirtazapine.
   b. Alpha-blockers (clonidine 0.1 mg bid or terazosin 1 to 2 mg qd)
6. For treatment of hot flashes related to menopausal symptoms in breast cancer patients
   a. Clonidine 0.1 mg q HS
   b. SSRIs/SNRIs: venlafaxine, paroxetine, escitalopram (fluoxetine and sertraline are no better than placebo)
   c. Gabapentin 300 mg tid (100 mg tid is no better than placebo)
   d. Complementary and alternative therapies have not shown effectiveness in controlled studies, including soy products/isoflavonones, evening primrose oil, dong quai, ginseng; there is no conclusive evidence for efficacy of acupuncture for this indication.
8. For prevention of macerated skin
   a. Zinc oxide paste applied to intertriginous areas and other at-risk sites

Goals/Outcomes

- Reduce fever, flushing, and diaphoresis-associated discomfort and distress
- Decrease sleep disruption
- Minimize caregiving burden

Documentation in the Medical Record

Initial Assessment

- Body temperature and associated signs and symptoms of fever
- Timing of fever, diaphoresis (day/night)
- Interventions (and results) attempted by caregiver
- Differential diagnosis based on history and physical examination

Interdisciplinary Progress Notes

- Effect of interventions on symptoms

IDT Care Plan

- Specific interventions and contingency plans

Recommended Reading

Adelson KB, Loprinzi CL, Hershman DL. Treatment of hot flushes in breast and prostate cancer. *Expert Opin Pharmacother* 2005; 6:1095–1110.

Calder K, Bruera E. Thalidomide for night sweats in patients with advanced cancer. *Palliat Med* 2000; 14:77–78.

Cowap J, Hardy J. Thioridazine in the management of cancer-related sweating. *J Pain Symptom Manage* 1998; 15:266.

Dodin S, Blanchet C, Marc I, et al. Acupuncture for menopausal hot flushes. *Cochrane Database Syst Rev* 2013, Issue 7. Art. No.: CD007410. DOI: 10.1002/14651858.CD007410.pub2.

Jeffery SM, Pepe JJ, Popovich LM, Vitigliano G. Gabapentin for hot flashes in prostate cancer. *Ann Pharmacother* 2002; 36:433–436.

Maida V. Nabilone for the treatment of paraneoplastic night sweats: a report of four cases. *J Palliat Med* 2008; 11(6):929–934.

Mercadante S. Hyoscine in opioid-induced sweating. *J Pain Symptom Manage* 1998; 15:214–215.

Meremikwu MM, Oyo-Ita A. Physical methods versus drug placebo or no treatment for managing fever in children. *Cochrane Database Syst Rev* 2003; 2. Art. No. CD004264.

Portzio G, Aielli F, Verna L, et al. Gabapentin in the treatment of severe sweating experienced by advanced cancer patients. *Support Care Cancer* 2006; 14:389–439.

Zylicz Z, Krajnik M. Flushing and sweating in an advanced breast cancer patient relieved by olanzapine. *J Pain Symptom Manage* 2003; 25:494–495.

Hiccups

SITUATION: Pain or discomfort and exhaustion due to persistent hiccups

Causes

- Gastric dysmotility with distention due to extrinsic obstruction or intrinsic disease
- Phrenic or vagus nerve irritation due to tumor or inflammation
- Alcohol ingestion
- Arrhythmia-induced syncope has been reported as both the cause and the effect of hiccups.
- Congenital malformations, malignancies, multiple sclerosis
- Cerebral neoplasms, metastasis or other CNS disorders (e.g., cerebrovascular disease)
- Recurrent laryngeal nerve irritation (mass lesions in neck, goiter, laryngitis)
- Metabolic disturbances (e.g., uremia, hypocalcemia, hyponatremia, fever, hypocarbia, hyperglycemia, hypokalemia)
- Medications: A wide variety of medications have been implicated in hiccups, including antibiotics, benzodiazepines, chemotherapeutics (e.g., cisplatin), corticosteroids (especially dexamethasone, although paradoxically

dexamethasone has been reported to relieve hiccups in AIDS-related progressive multifocal leukoencephalopathy, and other corticosteroids may relieve hiccups when dexamethasone may not), methyldopa, and opioids.

- Sepsis
- Reflux esophagitis
- Manifestation of anxiety disorder

Findings

- Disruption of social interactions, eating, sleeping
- "Heartburn" or other chest pain (from reflux or muscle strain)
- Aspiration-induced chronic cough, pneumonitis
- Anxiety, aerophagia

Assessment

Biomedical

- Systems review and physical examination for disease-related etiology as described earlier
- Metabolic evaluation
- Infection or tumor burden: Benefit versus burden of antibiotics or chemotherapy in patients where these interventions may be indicated for palliation should be decided among patient/family/IDT.
- Effect of hiccups on pain, sleep, significant fatigue, depression, and oral intake
- Association of hiccups with secondary disorders such as reflux and aspiration
- Determine relationship of hiccups episodes to position, medication use, and type of food intake.

Psychosocial

- Assess anxiety and "air swallowing" (aerophagia) as well as relationship of hiccups to sleep; hiccups that occur ONLY during wakefulness point to psychological causes.

Process of Care

Practical

- Nonpharmacological management techniques often suffice, but they may require repetition; these include various means of trying to stimulate nasopharyngeal reflexes and associated cranial nerves involved in the hiccup reflex arc. For instance:
  - Forcible traction on the tongue
  - Swallowing or applying granulated sugar under the tongue
  - Gargling with water, sipping ice water, biting on a lemon
  - Insertion of a small flexible catheter gently through the nose into the posterior pharynx
  - Elevating the uvula with a cotton-tipped applicator
  - Drinking from the far side of a glass (difficult for very ill patients to understand or carry out)
  - Cold application to the back of the neck

- Breathing into paper bag
- Elevating the head of the bed, or supporting patient in a semirecumbent position with pillows/bolsters, especially after meals
- Experimenting with position changes to determine if any one position offers relief (e.g., lateral)
- Acupuncture

Biomedical

- Adjunctive use of pharmacotherapy to maintain a "remission" from recurrent bouts of hiccups might be necessary. All of the following drug regimens have been found to be effective, but each patient requires a trial-and-error approach. Start with the therapy that is least toxic and least likely to induce side effects (this also depends on each patient's unique set of circumstances) and then try the next treatment on the list if needed:
  1. Chlorpromazine 25 to 50 mg IV (only FDA-approved medication for hiccups; effective in 80% of cases)
  2. Metoclopramide 10 to 20 mg PO/IV q8hr if there is delayed gastric emptying *without bowel obstruction*
  3. Simethicone and/or charcoal-containing antacids prn
  4. Haloperidol 1 to 5 mg PO/IV qid, or chlorpromazine 10 to 25 mg PO or 25-mg suppository PR qid
  5. Prednisone 1 mg/kg/day, then taper, if hepatomegaly or tumor effect is suspected as etiology
  6. Phenytoin 100 mg PO bid
  7. Valproic acid and carbamazepine have been effective when used in typical anticonvulsant doses.
  8. Gabapentin has been shown to be effective where CNS lesions are present and in some other etiologic groups, including in cancer patients.
  9. Baclofen, a centrally acting muscle relaxant, administered at 10 mg PO up to four times a day; particularly useful in patients for whom other agents are contraindicated (e.g., those with renal impairment)
  10. Proton-pump inhibitors may be useful if gastroesophageal reflux disease (GERD) or peptic ulcer disease is suspected to be a causative or contributing factor: omeprazole 20 mg PO daily for GERD or increase to 40 mg PO daily (20 mg PO twice daily for gastric or duodenal ulcers); lansoprazole 15 to 30 mg PO daily for GERD and duodenal or gastric ulcer
  11. Other drugs that have been successful based on case reports include edrophonium, corticosteroids, amantadine, nifedipine, and olanzapine.

Psychosocial

- Treat anxiety as described in "Agitation and Anxiety" earlier in this section.

Goals/Outcomes

- Reduce or eliminate episodes of hiccupping to the extent possible without incurring additional symptom burdens from treatment
- Provide periods of uninterrupted rest and sleep
- Improve social interaction and ability to partake of meals as per patient preference
- Eliminate "heartburn" and risk of aspiration

Documentation in the Medical Record

Initial Assessment

- Frequency and duration of hiccup episodes with inciting and relieving factors, if identified
- Putative etiology of hiccups, if identified
- Effect of hiccups on social interaction, meals, pain, sleep, mood

Interdisciplinary Progress Notes

- Effects of interventions

IDT Care Plan

- Decisions regarding value of further medical workup
- Specific interventions (nonmedical and medical) with contingency and follow-up plans

Recommended Reading

Marinella MA. Diagnosis and management of hiccups in the patient with advanced cancer. *J Support Oncol* 2009; 7(4):122–127.

Ong AM, Tan CS, Foo MW, Kee TY. Gabapentin for intractable hiccups in a patient undergoing peritoneal dialysis. *Perit Dial Int* 2008; 28(6):667–668.

Rizzo C, Vitale C, Montagnini M. Management of intractable hiccups: An illustrative case and review. *Am J Hosp Palliat Care* 2014; 31(2):220–224.

Turkyilmaz A, Eroglu A. Use of baclofen in the treatment of esophageal stent-related hiccups. *Ann Thorac Surg* 2008; 85(1):328–330.

Wilcox SK, Garry A, Johnson MJ. Novel use of amantadine: to treat hiccups. *J Pain Symptom Manage* 2009; 38(3):460–465.

Woelk CJ. Managing hiccups. *J Can Fam Physician* 2011; 57:672–675.

Imminent Death

SITUATION: Rapid decline in medical condition with associated signs and symptoms of imminent death

Findings

- Overall deterioration of bodily functions/homeostasis with accompanying general systems failure—all systems weaken
- Cardiac/progressive circulatory failure
  - Tachycardia that may degenerate to bradyarrhythmias
  - Hypotension
  - Weak peripheral pulses
  - Cool, mottled extremities
- GI
  - Disinterest in food
  - Dysphagia with liquids
- Renal insufficiency
  - Decreased urinary output

- Pulmonary failure
  - Tachypnea with periods of apnea (Cheyne-Stokes respirations)
  - Increased use of accessory muscles for respiration
  - Terminal congestion ("death rattle")
- Deterioration of cognition and higher brain functions/mental status changes
  - Progressive lethargy (obtundation)
  - Social withdrawal
  - Speaking to being(s) unseen by others in attendance
  - Picking at bedclothes or in the air
  - Agitation or restlessness

Assessment

- Assess the need for support by various members of the IDT, depending on areas of expertise, especially the need for spiritual and bereavement support.
- Anticipate the mode of death in order to prepare family/caregiver.
- Assess for behaviors suggestive of pain, dyspnea, fear.
- Determine whether bladder emptying is taking place.
  - Literature supports noninvasive bladder ultrasound as a new standard of care.
- Determine type of secretions causing "death rattle."
  - Oral: clear, relatively thin, not particularly malodorous
  - Bronchial: purulent, relatively thick, fetid odor
- Assess caregiver's level of comfort, capability, and competency with basic care (e.g., hygiene, positioning, medication administration).
- Determine if post-death plans have been made (funeral home, etc.).
- Review with caregiver whether important family members/significant others need to be or want to be notified of patient status.
- Determine whether current level of care is sufficient to manage patient symptoms and/or support caregiver.

Processes of Care

Practical and Biomedical

- Review and ensure provision of basic processes of physical care: oropharyngeal care (lips, teeth, oral mucosa), bathing, positioning, skin care, suctioning, medication administration.
- Ensure adequacy of urinary drainage, if urine is still being produced.
- Nonpurulent secretions: Patient's inability to control or swallow secretions often can be managed by positioning.
- Current literature base does not support the standard use of antimuscarininc drugs to treat death rattle. However, if the treating clinician believes that a trial of antimuscarinic medication is warranted, the choice of agent should be guided by convenience, cost, and likelihood of undesirable (adverse or toxic) effects. Appropriate monitoring and adjustments should be made based on response. Typical agents used include the following:
  1. Glycopyrrolate 0.2 mg IV/SQ prn (quaternary ammonium, does not cross blood–brain barrier)

2. Transdermal scopolamine patches: each patch delivers 1 mg of scopolamine per 24 hours for 3 days; more than one patch may be required, titrating therapeutic effects against potential side effects, which include sedation and delirium (tertiary amine, does cross blood–brain barrier and may cause CNS adverse side effects)

3. Hyoscyamine 0.125 mg SL q1–2hr prn (tertiary amine, does cross blood–brain barrier and may cause CNS adverse side effects)

4. Scopolamine 0.3 to 0.6 mg SQ prn (tertiary amine, does cross blood–brain barrier and may cause CNS adverse side effects)

5. Atropine 1 to 2 mg SQ/SL/nebulized q4hr or prn

- Purulent secretions should also be managed with positioning. Suctioning may be helpful in this situation.

- A single IV injection (if IV access is available) of a broad-spectrum antibiotic (e.g., a cephalosporin such as cefotaxime 500 to 1,000 mg IV) has been shown to decrease the bacterial count with accompanying elimination of malodorous character of bronchial secretions. This effect may last for days, allowing a much-reduced caregiving burden and eliminating a barrier to physical closeness. Furthermore, if pneumonia is thought to be present, then a full course of antibiotics may actually increase comfort.

- Restlessness or agitation: Refer to "Agitation and Anxiety" earlier in this section.

- Change route of medication administration if oral route has been in effect and this route is no longer feasible. Consult with physician/pharmacist as necessary for dosage conversions/formulations.

- Notify the primary care physician, as well as appropriate consulting physicians and/or hospice physician of status, depending on expressed preferences.

- Institute appropriate level of care to ensure adequate symptom management and essential care.

Psychosocial/Spiritual/Practical

- Continue to reassure patient through verbal communication and touch, even if there is no direct evidence of understanding or acknowledgment by the patient.

- Offer emotional support to caregiver, answer questions, and provide situation-specific information about processes of dying, including:
  - Possible occurrence of death during turning or other basic care
  - Possible occurrence of death during transport to another care facility if that becomes the choice/preference/necessity
  - Possible occurrence of a postmortem audible exhalation

- Help to distinguish and give reassurance to the caregiver and others in attendance about the difference between pain/suffering and terminal vocalizations, if present.

- Reassure caregiver/family that discontinuation of food/fluids when patient is no longer interested or responsive is "best care," reducing the burden to patient.

- Institute appropriate level of care to ensure adequate patient and caregiver support.

- Help to notify designated family, friends, clergy, etc., per patient/caregiver preferences.
- Review contingency plans for caregiver coping/support (e.g., 24-hour hospice telephone number in order to prevent a "panic" reaction such as dialing 911).
- Review information on procedure to follow after death, including disposition of body to funeral home or other prearrangements.
- Provide mouth and eye care: use toothette dipped in fluid of choice to moisten mouth and apply lip balm to keep lips from cracking; use artificial tears to moisten eyes, if open, and warm water and soft cloth to clear mucus/crusting.
- Facilitate and respect rituals as specified by patient/family.

Goals/Outcomes

- The dying process and death itself will occur with maximal comfort and with dignity
- Caregiver/family will experience a sense of enduring emotional comfort from the experience of their loved one dying in a nurturing/caring environment and in a manner that respected their preferences to the greatest extent possible

Documentation in the Medical Record

Initial Assessment

- Determination that on initial assessment the patient is imminently dying
- Focus of the evaluation should be on biomedical/psychosocial/practical/spiritual findings and preparation for death.

Interdisciplinary Progress Notes

- Ongoing and progressive physical signs and symptoms
- Coping by caregiver/family
- Description of instructions, preparations, interventions
- Results of interventions

IDT Care Plan

- Specific interventions planned
- Contingency plans and schedule of follow-up by various members of IDT
- Updated bereavement plan

Recommended Reading

Currow DC, Abernethy AP. Respiratory problems. *Curr Opin Support Palliat Care* 2009; 3(2):120–124.

Hui D, Dos Santos R, Chisholm G, et al. Bedside clinical signs associated with impending death in patients with advanced cancer: preliminary findings of a prospective, longitudinal, cohort study. *Cancer* 2015; 121(6):960–967.

Hui D, Dos Santos R, Chisholm G, et al. Clinical signs of impending death in cancer patients. *Oncologist* 2014; 19:681–687.

Lokker ME, Van Zuylen L, Van der Rijit CCD, Van der Heide A. Prevalence, impact and treatment of death rattle: a systematic review. *J Pain Symptom Manage* 2014; 47:105–122.

Muir JC, von Gunten CF. Antisecretory agents in gastrointestinal obstruction. *Clin Geriatr Med* 2000; 16(2):327–334.

Newman DK, Gaines T, Snare E. Innovation in bladder assessment: use of technology in extended care. *J Gerontol Nurs* 2005; 31(12):33–41.

Shimizu Y, Miyashita M, Morita T, et al. Care strategy for death rattle in terminally ill cancer patients and their family members: recommendations from a cross-sectional nationwide survey of bereaved family members' perceptions. *J Pain Symptom Manage* 2014; 48(1):2–12.

Van der Steen JT, Ooms ME, van der Wal G, Ribbe MW. Pneumonia: the demented patient's best friend? Discomfort after starting or withholding antibiotic treatment. *J Am Geriatr Soc* 2002; 50:1681–1688.

Wildiers H, Demeulenaere P, Clement P, Menten J. Treatment of death rattle in dying patients. *Belgian J Med Oncol* 2008; 2:275–279.

Insomnia and Nocturnal Restlessness

SITUATION: Disturbed sleep or significant alteration in sleep pattern interfering with patient sense of well-being or adding to caregiver burden

Sleep disorders are common in the general population, and many studies indicate they are even more frequent in hospice and palliative care patients. Sleep disorders may be described by patients as delayed onset of sleep (increased sleep latency), difficulty maintaining sleep, early awakening, or a combination of these disturbances.

Although sleep problems are common in the hospice and palliative care patient population, they may be underreported and underrecognized in these patients for a variety of reasons. Patients may believe sleep problems are inevitable or unavoidable concomitants of serious illness, or believe that their sleep symptoms are inconsequential compared to the severity of their chronic, progressive disease. In addition, patients with cognitive or communication impairments may not be able to report their sleep symptoms. Poor sleep has a great impact on mood, coping abilities, pain tolerance, interpersonal relations, appetite, energy, and overall sense of well-being. It is therefore important to regularly inquire of patients and caregivers whether patients are experiencing problems with sleep.

Causes

Biomedical

- Physical symptoms and dysfunctions may contribute to sleep disturbances:
  - Pain
  - Urinary retention
  - Constipation
  - Dyspnea
  - Heartburn

- Nausea
- Pruritus
- Diarrhea
- Urinary frequency
- Abdominal distention from ascites or tumor burden
- A preexisting sleep disorder may continue to cause symptoms and may be worsened by the illness or therapy; obstructive and central sleep apnea may be worsened by prescribed opioids, anticholinergics, or benzodiazepines.
- CNS-stimulating agents (e.g., caffeine, nicotine) and medications may disturb sleep (e.g., decongestants, methylxanthines, SSRIs, psychostimulants, corticosteroids); opioids prescribed for pain may cause daytime somnolence and thereby interfere with nighttime sleep.
- Chemotherapy and radiation therapy are associated with daytime fatigue and disrupted nighttime sleep patterns.
- Use of illicit drugs, alcohol, or tobacco or withdrawal from these substances may disrupt normal sleep patterns.

Psychosocial/Spiritual

- Emotional, psychological, or spiritual concerns may cause nighttime rumination and worry and may impair sleep.

Practical/Environmental

- Environmental factors in the living area may impair sound sleep (e.g., noisy equipment such as oxygen concentrators; nighttime caregiving needs that awaken the patient; an uncomfortable bed; intrusive catheters, SQ or IV lines).
- Inadequate sleep hygiene: Good sleep hygiene practices normally include reserving the bedroom and bed for intimate activities and sleep only; as patients become weaker, however, they may spend the majority of the day and perform their daily activities (reading, watching television, listening to music) in the bedroom and in bed; they can no longer adhere to this component of good sleep hygiene.
- Recent hospitalization: In the hospital, patients' sleep is often interrupted by patient care activities and bright lights during the night. This disturbs the normal sleep–wake cycle, and when patients return home, they often have trouble reestablishing their previous sleep patterns.

Findings

- Complaint of poor sleep, exhaustion (by patient and/or caregiver, family members)
- Cognitively functional and expressive patients may be able to report on sleep history, but many patients are not aware of the details of sleep disturbance or nocturnal behaviors, requiring reliance on caregiver reports and/or daytime symptoms.
- Moodiness, grouchiness, emotional lability/volatility
- Daytime sedation, nighttime restlessness
- Caregiver fatigue, frustration, exasperation, depression

Assessment

Biomedical

- Sleep history
  - Onset of sleep, frequency of wakening, total duration, daytime sleep; use sleep assessment questionnaires (Pittsburgh Sleep Quality Index; Epworth Sleepiness Scale) and/or sleep diaries (National Sleep Foundation), if appropriate
- Assess for inadequately treated symptoms of primary and related disease processes, especially pain and dyspnea (orthopnea).
- Evaluate for signs or symptoms of primary sleep disorder (restless legs syndrome, other movement disorder, obstructive sleep apnea, night terrors).
- Review prescribed medications and treatments and evaluate their effect on sleep.
- Review use of alcohol, tobacco, nonprescribed medications, and illicit medications and substances whose use may have increased or decreased.
- Explore how the sleep disorder is affecting patient/caregiver function.

Psychosocial/Spiritual

- Explore emotional, psychological, social, and spiritual concerns and distress that may impair sleep.
- Get corroboration of sleep pattern from others in home (especially if patient has impaired cognition or communication).
- Determine patient and caregiver expectations of acceptable sleep pattern.
- Assess caregiver fatigue and coping strategies.

Practical

- Assess sleeping area and environmental factors (bed and bedding/pillows, noise, temperature, privacy).
- Assess safety if patient is up at night (nightlight, proximity of commode, obstacles, etc.).

Processes of Care

Practical/Psychosocial/Spiritual

- Progressive relaxation techniques/exercises as appropriate
- Small carbohydrate bedtime snack/beverage (e.g., warm milk with favorite flavoring)
- Pre-sleep talk, storytelling, music
- Ensure a safe environment.
- Maximize daytime activities and stimulation (use of volunteers, etc.).
- Components of sleep hygiene (some of these measures may not be applicable to a debilitated, bed-bound patient)
  — Maintain a regular sleep routine.
  — Avoid naps if possible.
  — Do not stay in bed awake for more than 5 to 10 minutes.
  — Do not drink caffeine late in the day.
  — Do not watch television in bed or read in bed.

— Avoid substances that interfere with sleep.
— Exercise regularly (if possible).
— Have a quiet, comfortable bedroom.
— If patient is a "clock watcher" at night, hide the clock.
— Have a comfortable pre-bedtime routine.
— Consider sleep restriction. For patients who are not bed-bound, encourage them to stay in bed for only the number of hours that they are able to sleep. If unable to sleep they should get out of bed and engage in a quiet relaxing activity until sleepy again. Patient should retire to bed 15 minutes earlier every night until the preferred sleep duration is achieved.

• Increase level of care if caregiver exhaustion or inadequate coping.
• Supportive counseling for mood disturbance (anxiety, depression)
  • Facilitate expression of fears, worries, "unfinished business."

Biomedical

• Optimize medical management of contributing causes of pain, dyspnea, hypoxia, urinary frequency, GERD, etc.
• Evaluate and treat or mitigate primary sleep disorders (obstructive sleep apnea, restless legs syndrome).
  • Symptomatic management of restless legs
    — Low-dose sedating TCA (e.g., amitriptyline 10 mg PO q HS)
    — Low-dose Sinemet (carbidopa/levodopa; initial dose 10 mg PO q HS)
    — Gabapentin (initial dose 100 mg PO q HS)
    — Ropinirole (initial dose 0.25 mg PO q HS)
• Adjust medication schedule to the extent feasible to eliminate daytime sedation and nocturnal stimulation.
• Treat anxiety, depression if not responsive to nonpharmacological interventions.
• Advise and educate patient about hazards of illicit substance use, alcohol and tobacco use, or recent reduction in use, and over-the-counter medication use.
• Pharmacotherapy
  NOTE: There is a risk of increasing confusion, obtundation, daytime sedation, balance disturbances, etc., with the addition of any CNS depressant, especially in the frail elderly; close monitoring and low-dose titration are important. A short trial of medication (e.g., 2 weeks) is preferable if insomnia is causing considerable distress and while nonpharmacological and symptom-driven therapies are commenced.
  • Benzodiazepines: These medications decrease the time to sleep onset and prolong the first and second stages of sleep. Short- or medium-acting agents are preferred because they minimize daytime sleepiness and are less likely to cause complex sleep-related behaviors. Most benzodiazepines interact with inhibitors of CYP3A4 such as macrolide antibiotics; concurrent administration with CYP3A4 inhibitors or with alcohol or other CNS depressants, including certain opioids (e.g., fentanyl) may increase the CNS depressant effects of benzodiazepines.
    • Short-acting agents: triazolam 0.125 to 0.25 mg; oxazepam 10 to 30 mg

- Intermediate-acting agents: estazolam 1 to 2 mg; lorazepam 1 to 5 mg; temazepam 15 to 30 mg
- Benzodiazepine receptor agonists: zaleplon (ultrashort-acting) 5 to 20 mg; zolpidem (short-acting) 5 to 10 mg; eszopiclone (intermediate duration) 1 to 3 mg
- Melatonin receptor agonists: ramelteon (short-acting) 8 mg (avoid administration with a high-fat meal)
- Sedating antidepressants
  - These agents can be used for sleep due to significant sedating effects; anticholinergic effects must be carefully monitored: amitriptyline 10 to 25 mg PO q HS (titrate as needed); doxepin 10 to 25 mg PO q HS (titrate as needed); trazodone 25 to 50 mg PO q HS (titrate as needed); mirtazapine 15 to 45 mg PO q HS
- Antihistamines
  - This class of agents is best avoided due to anticholinergic side effects such as dry mouth and urinary retention; in addition they may cause mental clouding and ataxia, particularly in elderly patients.
- Alcohol
  - Patients may use alcohol to induce sleep, but this should be discouraged: alcohol initially induces CNS depression and sleep, but it can cause rebound excitation and insomnia. In addition, alcohol may provoke gastroesophageal reflux and may have a diuretic effect, both of which can disrupt sleep.
- Natural and herbal remedies
  - There are no clearly proven remedies in this category; the purity and optimal dose of these remedies have not been established.
- Nocturnal delirium ("sundowning")
  - If nocturnal delirium is suspected, precipitating factors should be promptly sought and treated.
  - Consider the possibility that alcohol or drug withdrawal may be producing the symptoms; patients may need treatment for withdrawal syndrome.
  - While reversible medical causes are being assessed and treated, behavioral interventions should begin:
    — Patients should have a predictable routine.
    — Extraneous stimuli should be minimized.
    — Lighting should be improved to reduce confusion and allow patients who may have impaired sight to see familiar surroundings.
    — Ensure safety of the environment.
    — Ensure (when patient's physical status permits) adequate food and fluid.
    — Assess for presence of urinary retention or constipation.
    — Provide for dry clothing and adequate warmth or coolness.
    — Constantly reassure and reorient.
  - For nocturnal delirium/agitation not responsive to nonpharmacological treatments, low doses of antipsychotic agents may be helpful: chlorpromazine 25 mg PO q HS; haloperidol 0.5 to 2 mg PO q HS; risperidone 0.25 to 2 mg PO daily

Goals/Outcomes

- Normalize patient sleep patterns
- Relieve distressing nocturnal symptoms
- Relieve caregiver burden during nocturnal hours

Documentation in the Medical Record

Initial Assessment

- Sleep patterns and symptoms of disturbed sleep
- Evaluation of causative factors
- Medication review
- Impact of sleep disturbance on patient and caregiver
- Interventions
- Effectiveness of interventions

Interdisciplinary Progress Notes

- Ongoing identification of contributing factors
- Results of interventions and adjustment of care plan

IDT Care Plan

- Nonpharmacological and pharmacological interventions
- Psychological, social, spiritual supports offered
- Prevention of caregiver burnout
- Plans for patient safety

Recommended Reading

Mercadante S, Aielli F, Asile C, et al. Sleep disturbances in patients with advanced cancer in different palliative care settings. *J Pain Symptom Manage* 2015; 50(6):786–792.

Renom-Guiteras A, Planas J, Farriois C, et al. Insomnia among patients with advanced disease during admission in a palliative care unit: a prospective observational study on its frequency and association with psychological, physical and environmental factors. *BMC Palliative Care* 2014; 13:40.

Staedt J, Stoppe G. Treatment of rest-activity disorders in dementia and special focus on sundowning. *Int J Geriatric Psychiatry* 2005; 20(6):507–511.

Volicer L, Harper D, Manning B, et al. Sundowning and circadian rhythms in Alzheimer's disease. *Am J Psychiatry* 2001; 158:704–711.

Nausea and Vomiting

SITUATION: Recurrent or chronic nausea and/or vomiting

Definitions and Physiology

- **Acute nausea and vomiting:** occurs within 24 hours of event (e.g., chemotherapy/eating)
- **Delayed nausea and vomiting:** occurs more than 24 hours after chemotherapy

- **Anticipatory nausea and vomiting:** occurs before a new cycle of chemotherapy/event due to sensory conditioned stimuli (e.g., odor, sound, sight)
- **Breakthrough nausea and vomiting:** occurs within 5 days of prophylactic use of antivomiting medication and requires additional dose

The physiology of nausea and vomiting involves multiple areas, neurotransmitters, pathways, and targets within the CNS and periphery that ultimately trigger activity in the vomiting center of the brain. These include the chemoreceptor trigger zone (CTZ), which involves dopamine, serotonin, and neurokinin; the cortex, which involves acetylcholine, serotonin, and histamine; peripheral pathways, which involve serotonin, norepinephrine, and acetylcholine; and vestibular activation, which involves acetylcholine and histamine. The complexity of this "system" allows for activation by a wide variety of mechanical and chemical stimuli, but conversely it also allows therapeutic intercession by a wide variety of agents.

Causes

Biomedical

- Visceral or GI tract disorders (e.g., malignancy, bowel obstruction, ileus, constipation)
- CNS disturbances (e.g., neoplasm, increased intracranial pressure)
- Chemical triggers (e.g., odors, tastes, drugs [especially chemotherapy])
- Vestibular disturbances
- Metabolic disturbances (e.g., hypercalcemia, hyperglycemia, uremia, infection)
- Mechanical triggers (e.g., gagging from coughing, hiccuping, retained secretions)

Psychosocial

- Conditioned response to situational/environmental/emotional/sensory stimuli
- Anxiety related to anticipation of nausea and/or vomiting

Findings

Biomedical

- Continuous or episodic nausea with or without vomiting
- Passive or projectile vomiting independent of or associated with food/fluid or medication intake

Psychosocial

- Varying degrees of withdrawal, fatigue, depressed mood, anxiety, aversion to triggering factors
- Varying degrees of acceptance, frustration, aversion by caregiver

Assessment

Biomedical

- Systems review and physical examination to assess for:
  - Distention, bloating, evidence of bowel obstruction, peptic ulcer/gastritis/esophagitis, severe constipation or impaction
  - Hepatomegaly

- Evidence of elevated intracranial pressure (papilledema, headache, altered mental status, spontaneous projectile vomiting)
- Dehydration
- Oropharyngeal examination (dentures, thrush, hyperreactive gag reflex)
- Medication review with attention to emetogenic or irritant drugs such as chemotherapy agents, opioids, digoxin, theophylline, NSAIDs
- Frequency, volume, color (e.g., bilious), odor (e.g., feculent), consistency (digested/undigested) of vomitus
- Relationship of nausea/vomiting to any specific recurrent activity, event, position, etc.
- Chemotherapy agents with high nausea effects (documented in more than 90% of patients): cisplatin, mechlorethamine, cisplatin streptozotocin, cyclophosphamide (in doses greater than 1,500 mg/m^2), carmustine, dacarbazine, dactinomycin
- Chemotherapy agents with moderate nausea effects (documented in 30% to 90% of patients): carboplatin, cyclophosphamide (in doses less than 1,500 mg/m^2), daunorubicin, doxorubicin, epirubicin, idarubicin, oxaliplatin, cytarabine, ifosfamide, irinotecan

Psychosocial

- Effect of symptoms on mood, energy, social interaction, interest in activities
- Relationship of symptoms to psychological causes
- Effect of vomiting on caregiver coping

Processes of Care

Practical

- Reduce odors and place visual stimuli that trigger nausea/vomiting out of direct eyesight.
- Optimize air circulation.
- Have ample supply of fresh cold water for mouth rinsing and to apply to back of neck and brow.
- Institute appropriate level of care in order to implement indicated symptom management and support.
- Minimize oral intake to the degree preferred by the patient; reinstitute clear liquids as desired after 24 hours of relief from vomiting. Discontinue all oral intake if bowel obstruction is suspected or confirmed.

Biomedical

- Basic principles
  1. Obviate and treat the underlying cause whenever possible.
  2. Prevention is more successful than treatment.
     - Administer antiemetic prior to known triggers of nausea/vomiting.
  3. Use nonpharmacological approaches whenever possible:
     - Acupuncture/acupressure
     - Relaxation techniques/foot massage/herbs/ginger
  4. The oral route is preferred for prophylactic pharmacotherapy.
  5. Use the rectal or parenteral (e.g., SQ) route to initiate treatment for the first 24 to 48 hours to control symptoms; then convert to the oral route if possible.

6. Use combination therapies of mechanistically different agents without similar toxicities for intractable symptoms.

- Pharmacotherapy specific for nausea/vomiting due to:
  1. Delayed gastric emptying/impaired GI motility
     a. Metoclopramide 10 to 20 mg PO q6–8hr; 1 to 2 mg/hr SQ infusion
     b. Add simethicone/charcoal to decrease gas, if eructation is present.
     c. Decrease intrinsic and extrinsic abdominal pressure: Elevate head of bed, use loose-fitting and nonbinding clothing.
  2. Initiation or escalation of therapy
     a. Metoclopramide (dopamine receptors) 10 to 20 mg PO q6–8hr; 1 to 2 mg/hr SQ infusion
     b. Diphenhydramine (histamine receptors) 25 to 50 mg PO q6–8hr
     c. Prochlorperazine (dopamine receptors) 25 mg PR or trimethobenzamide 200 mg PR q6hr

- Reassess in 3 to 4 days; tolerance to nausea and emetogenic effects of opioids usually occurs, allowing discontinuation of these antiemetic drugs. If nausea and/or vomiting continue(s), assess for other causes prior to changing analgesic.
  3. Bowel obstruction (nonsurgical care in terminal stage of disease)
     a. Octreotide 150 µg deep SQ (intrafat) 12 hr or 300 µg/24 hr continuous SQ infusion, combined with opioid analgesic, titrated to effect
     b. Nasogastric suctioning only if necessary, feasible, low bleeding risk (i.e., thrombocytopenia) and tolerated
  4. Vestibular disturbance: meclizine 25 mg PO bid
  5. Vagal stimulation (bowel obstruction, hepatic capsular pressure, thrush): scopolamine 0.3 to 0.6 mg SQ prn (monitor for psychotomimetic effects)
  6. Increased intracranial pressure (brain tumor or metastasis): dexamethasone 4 mg q8hr and increase as necessary to control symptoms
  7. Metabolic abnormalities (hypercalcemia, uremia): haloperidol 0.5 mg q6–8hr

- Nonspecific and adjunctive therapy
  1. The use of dopamine receptor antagonists (e.g., haloperidol 0.5 to 2 mg PO/IV q6hr prn or prochlorperazine 10 to 25 mg PO/25 to 100 mg PR q6hr prn) in patients who can tolerate the sedating effects is generally effective as primary or adjunctive therapy for most causes of severe nausea and vomiting. **These agents are contraindicated in patients with Parkinson's disease.**
  2. The addition of lorazepam 0.5 to 2 mg SL/IV may be useful as an adjunctive agent for control of nausea associated with many etiologies, or when there are nonspecified causes.
  3. Dexamethasone is frequently used in the prevention and treatment of chemotherapy- and radiation therapy–induced nausea and vomiting, as an adjunctive therapy with dopamine receptor antagonists, benzodiazepines, and/or serotonin 5-HT$_3$ receptor blockers. Dexamethasone 6 to 16 mg has cited to help with nausea and vomiting in bowel obstruction.
  4. Ondansetron (4 to 8 mg IV/PO q6–12hr), granisetron (1 to 2 mg PO q12hr [available as tablets and oral solution 1 mg/5 ml] or 10 µg/kg), and dolasetron (100 mg PO or 1.8 mg/kg IV) are 5-HT$_3$ receptor blockers

that have been used for control of nausea and vomiting associated with chemotherapy and certain postoperative circumstances. The newest of these agents, palonosetron, is the most potent and is recommended only as a single 0.25-mg IV dose. These drugs should be considered in those cases resistant to therapies listed earlier. Ondansetron binds to dopamine, serotonin, alpha-1, cholinergic (muscarinic), and histamine receptors.

5. Aprepitant (125 mg PO followed by 80 mg PO qd) is a substance P antagonist and may be used in conjunction with other antiemetics for refractory nausea/vomiting resulting from oncologic therapies. It has also been studied to help with gastroparesis.

6. Olanzapine (2.5 mg PO daily titrating to 7.5 mg daily over 7 to 10 days as needed) is an "atypical" antipsychotic medication of the thienbenzodiazepine class that blocks multiple emetogenic neurotransmitters, including those affecting the following receptors: dopamine, serotonin, alpha-1 adrenergic, acetylcholine (muscarinic), and histamine. This may provide benefit when multiple emetogenic pathways are involved.

7. Dronabinol (5 to 10 mg PO/PR q6–8hr) can provide relief from nausea by selective binding at cannabinoid receptors (CB1, CB2). In addition, anxiolytic effects have been attributed to this synthetic cannabinoid that may be beneficial in cases of anticipatory nausea.

Psychosocial

- Use imaging and relaxation techniques to control anxiety or apprehension associated with or causing nausea/vomiting.
- Teach caregiver management techniques to minimize stress and burden to the extent possible.

Goals/Outcomes

- Minimize nausea
- Decrease episodes of vomiting to a maximum of one or two episodes per day
- Reduce care burden
- Reduce social isolation brought on by intractable nausea and vomiting

Documentation in the Medical Record

Initial Assessment

- Frequency and characteristics of nausea/vomiting episodes
- Likely etiology and/or associated causative factors (e.g., food, constipation, opioids, smells, medications, portion/spoon size, movement)
- Nutritional/hydration status
- Emotional/psychological status: mood, sleep, social interaction, energy
- Physical findings: oropharyngeal and abdominal examination, skin turgor, activity level
- Coping ability of caregiver around this symptom complex

Interdisciplinary Progress Notes

- Description, sequence, and timing of interventions attempted
- Results of interventions, including adverse effects (if any) of pharmacotherapy

- Emotional and physical findings from follow-up visits; caregiver capabilities and coping

IDT Care Plan

- Timing, sequence, and types of interventions
- Schedule of follow-up visits and contingency plans (assessment for additional support for refractory symptoms: continuous care or higher level of care [inpatient unit])

Recommended Reading

Ernst E, Pittler MH. Efficacy of ginger for nausea and vomiting: A systematic review of randomized clinical trials. *Br J Anesthesia* 2000; 84(3):367–371.

Fahler J, Wall GC, Leman BI. Gastroparesis-associated refractory nausea treated with aprepitant. *Ann Pharmacother* 2012; 46(12):e38.

Genç F, Tan M. The effect of acupressure application on chemotherapy-induced nausea, vomiting, and anxiety in patients with breast cancer. *Palliat Support Care* 2015; 13(2):275–284.

Glare PA, Dunwoodie D, Clark K, et al. Treatment of nausea and vomiting in terminally ill cancer patients. *Drugs* 2008; 68(18):2575–2590.

Henzi I, Walder B, Tramer M. Dexamethasone for the prevention of postoperative nausea and vomiting: a quantitative systematic review. *Anesth Analg* 2000; 90(1):186–194.

MacKintosh D. Olanzapine in the management of difficult to control nausea and vomiting in a palliative care population: a case series. *J Palliat Med* 2016; 19(1):87–90.

PDQ Supportive and Palliative Care Editorial Board. Nausea and vomiting. Published online September 2, 2015. Available at http://www.ncbi.nlm.nih.gov/pubmedhealth/PMH0032557/.

Tramer MR, Carroll D, Campbell F, et al. Cannabinoids for control of chemotherapy-induced nausea and vomiting: A quantitative systematic review. *Br Med J* 2001; 323:1–6.

Pain

SITUATION: Continuous and/or intermittent pain—defined as an unpleasant sensory and emotional experience—that interferes with basic functions, activities, sleep, or social interaction, or otherwise erodes the patient's quality of life to any meaningful extent

Pain is a very common symptom in cancer and other chronic progressive disease states. Along with severe anxiety/agitation/delirium and dyspnea, pain that is out of control represents one of the urgent/emergent symptom complexes encountered in the hospice setting. Pain assessment, establishment of patient goals, and treatment plans should be put into place as a high priority and can be best achieved with an understanding that pain is a highly personal experience, modified and amplified by past experience; immediate psychological, physical, and social context; future expectations; cultural norms; and spiritual orientation. Preventive approaches to pain management, rapid responses by the team to calls for help when pain is out of control, and the ability to intervene effectively in a timely manner are key and fundamental measures of quality hospice care.

Causes

Biomedical

- Basic principle: Identify the cause of pain, and treat with the most appropriate intervention:
  1. Cancer-related: pain associated with direct or metastatic tumor involvement of bone, nerves, viscera, or soft tissues (60% to 80% of all cancer patients)
  2. Cancer treatment-related: pain associated with antineoplastic therapy (20% to 25% of cancer patients), including surgery, radiation therapy (early and late effects), and chemotherapy
  3. Other common painful disorders associated with advanced disease states:
     a. Somatic: musculoskeletal damage (e.g., arthropathies, spine facet disease, and myofascial pain), skin and mucosal ulceration, cervicogenic headache
     b. Visceral: ischemic, GI and genitourinary insults (e.g., myocardial infarction, fecal and/or urinary retention, bowel obstruction)
     c. Neuropathic: centrally mediated (such as post-stroke pain, parkinsonism, phantom limb pain, post-herpetic neuralgia), peripherally mediated (e.g., HIV, diabetes, peripheral vascular disease), and less well-understood chronic pain syndromes (e.g., post-laminectomy pain; migraine/cluster headache)

Psychosocial/Spiritual

- Basic principle: Any amount of pain can lead to a lot of suffering, and any amount of suffering can greatly amplify the pain experience.
  1. Pain due to any disease is often greatly amplified by interpersonal conflict or unresolved intrapersonal issues (psychological or spiritual), especially when the pain is a constant reminder of the seriousness of the illness.
  2. Pain, anxiety, and depression reinforce each other as complex psychophysiological interactions that often cannot be readily separated. Detailed assessment is necessary in order to direct therapy in the most specific and efficacious way.

Findings

Biomedical

- Patient report of pain/discomfort
- Facial expressions or body posturing suggestive of pain (e.g., grimacing, guarding)
- Vocalizations suggestive of pain
- Tachycardia, tachypnea, hypertension, diaphoresis

NOTE: Absence of these autonomic findings does not rule out pain; presence of these findings in a non–self-reporting patient is suggestive, especially when repositioning, performing personal cares, dressing changes, etc.

Psychosocial

- Functional impairment (impacting work, school, or home-based tasks)
- Poor sleep
- Decreased coping
- Agitation/restlessness; emotional volatility (ill-tempered; "short fuse")
- Withdrawal from social interaction
- Decreased interest in previous enjoyments (e.g., television viewing, reading, sewing, etc.)
- Reluctance to participate in life review
- Signs/symptoms of depression, anxiety
- Reduced appetite, decreased interest in food, and/or altered eating patterns

Assessment

Biomedical and Psychosocial/Spiritual

- Basic principle: Believe the patient's report of pain. Because pain is a subjective phenomenon, the caregiver/clinician must believe that the patient's report of pain is real. Objective physiological indicators of acute pain such as tachycardia, sweating, pallor, or affective responses such as facial grimacing are helpful when present but are often absent when pain is chronic or continuous (Fig. 3.1).
- Take a careful history, using mnemonic "OPQRST":
  1. O for Onset (when did it/does it start?)
  2. P for Pain gets better with . . ./gets worse with . . .
  3. Q for Quality (e.g., burning, achy, etc.)
  4. R for Radiation (e.g., where does it start and where does it spread?)
  5. S for Severity
     a. Use validated pain rating scales (Fig. 3.2) or the Edmonton Symptom Assessment System (ESAS); see http://www.npcrc.org/files/news/edmonton_symptom_assessment_scale.pdf for patients who can self-report.
     b. Use PAIN AD (Table 3.1) for non–self-reporting patients.
  6. T for Temporal Course
     a. Constant or episodic pattern
     b. When is the pain most severe?
     c. Breakthrough pain: frequency, severity, and duration
        i. Incident pain (caused by specific activity or action)
        ii. Spontaneous pain (no identifiable cause)
        iii. End-of-dose failure (pain returns before next dose of regularly scheduled medicine takes effect)
     d. Use of a 24-hour pain diary in an able patient, or completed by a caregiver, helps to identify many factors and effects of interventions (Fig. 3.3; make copies for patient/caregiver as needed).

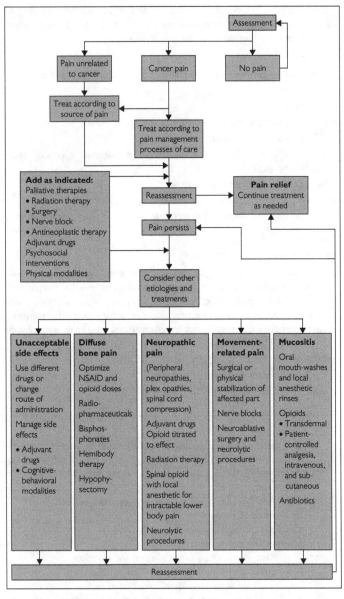

Figure 3.1 Flow chart for continuing evaluation and treatment of pain. Adapted from AHCPR Clinical Guideline Number 9.

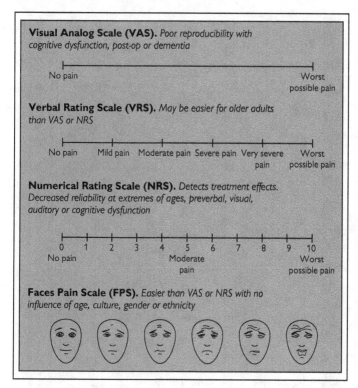

Figure 3.2 Unidimensional pain scale. Reprinted from *The Journal of Pain*, May;41(2). Bieri D, Reeve RA, Champion GD, Addicoat L, Ziegler JB. The Faces Pain Scale for the self-assessment of the severity of pain experienced by children: Development, initial validation, and preliminary investigation for ratio scale properties, pp. 139–150, © 1990 with permission from Elsevier.

- Assess the effect of pain on the patient's mood, activities of daily living (ADLs), sleep, appetite, movement, toileting, social interactions, interest in life, and previous enjoyments.
- Take a careful analgesic history, including prior and present medications, analgesic response (time to onset of meaningful pain relief and duration of action), and undesirable or adverse effects, including frank allergies and GI upset.
- Perform physical examination and review systems specific to pain complaints.
- Review and consider necessity for corroborating diagnostic testing only if the diagnosis is in question or treatment/care plan will be meaningfully affected (e.g., radiograph for suspected pathological fracture).
- Treat pain empirically while evaluation is being completed.

Table 3.1 Pain Assessment in Advanced Dementia: PAIN-AD Scale

	0	1	2	Score
Breathing Independent of Vocalization	Normal	Occasional labored breathing Short period of hyperventilation	Noisy labored breathing Long period of hyperventilation Cheyne-Stokes respirations	
Negative Vocalization	None	Occasional moan or groan Low-level speech with a negative or disapproving quality	Repeated troubled calling out Loud moaning or groaning Crying	
Facial Expression	Smiling or inexpressive	Sad Frightened Frown	Facial grimacing	
Body Language	Relaxed	Tense Distressed pacing Fidgeting	Rigid Fists clenched Knees pulled up Pulling or pushing away Striking out	
Consolability	No need to console	Distracted or reassured by voice or touch	Unable to console, distract or reassure	

Adapted from Warden V, Hurley AC, Volicer L. Development and psychometric evaluation of the Pain Assessment in Advanced Dementia (PAINAD) scale. *J Am Med Dir Assoc* 2003; 4(1):9–15.

Notes on the PAIN-AD Scale:

Scoring: The total score ranges from 0–10 points. 1–3=mild pain; 4–6=moderate pain; 7–10=severe pain. These ranges are based on a standard 0–10 scale of pain.

It is to be completed after the patient is observed for at least 5 minutes, under any circumstance (such as at rest, during caregiving, or after administration of pain medication).

PAIN-AD scoring may be confounded by the following scored symptoms which may actually be due to non-painful situations: Cheyne-Stokes respirations (score of 2 points for breathing), which may be due to imminent death, and flexion contractures (score of 2 points for body language), which may be due to end-stage dementia.

Twenty-four Hour Pain Diary

Patient Name:_____ Date:_____

Time	Maximal Pain 0–10 scale	Minimal Pain 0–10 scale	Medication: name, dose, route of administration	Activities: lying, sitting, walking, eating, toilet, etc.
12 Midnight				
1 am				
2				
3				
4				
5				
6				
7				
8				
9				
10				
11				
12 Noon				
1 pm				
2				
3				
4				
5				
6				
7				
8				
9				
10				
11				

Figure 3.3 Twenty-four-hour pain diary.

- Be as specific as possible in determining the cause of the pain whenever possible (e.g., fecal impaction, bowel obstruction, epidural metastasis, plexopathy, lytic bone lesion, etc.) and institute diagnosis-specific therapy immediately.
- Evaluate level of anxiety and signs of depressive mood disorder.
- Evaluate for contributors to pain/suffering of a psychological/spiritual nature (e.g., guilt, punishment, abandonment by God, etc.).
- Evaluate patient/caregiver understanding and use of analgesics as well as non-pharmacological pain-reducing interventions (e.g., relaxation, imaging, meditation, massage, heat, cooling, music, etc.), including importance of pretreatment (30 to 60 minutes for oral medications) before a predictably pain-producing event or activity (e.g., personal care, transfers, dressing changes, etc.).
- Reevaluate pain complaints and effects of interventions at least daily, or more frequently as dictated by individual circumstances.

- Determine appropriate level of care, based on patient/caregiver response to therapies and coping abilities.
- Barriers to good pain management
  - Discounting a patient's subjective measure of pain
  - Difficulty in assessment of the cognitively impaired
  - Practitioner, patient, and caregiver fears about opioid therapy, including excessive concerns of addiction and hastening death
- Patients need to be educated about medication adherence (use specifically and only as directed), physical versus psychological dependence, tolerance, the disease of addiction, side effects, and appropriate dosing of analgesics. Many patients as well as family members believe the use of opioids, regardless of indications, will inevitably lead to addiction, creating a deep-seated reluctance to use opioids for analgesia.

Teaching Points

- All opioids will result in physical dependence after a few weeks of use, and sudden discontinuation should be avoided as this may cause symptoms of withdrawal.
- Physical dependence is not addiction.
- **Addiction** is a primary, chronic neurobiological disease characterized by behaviors that include impaired control over drug use, craving, compulsive use, and continued use despite harm.
- **Pseudo-addiction** may occur when there is inadequate pain control, leading to desperate-appearing behaviors suggestive of "drug seeking"—however, patients are, in fact, "pain relief seeking." Aberrant behaviors around medication use require a differential diagnosis to determine the underlying cause.
- **Physical dependence** is a state of adaptation that is manifested by a drug class–specific withdrawal syndrome that can be produced by abrupt cessation, rapid dose reduction, decreasing blood level of the drug, and/or administration of an antagonist.
- **Tolerance** is a state of adaptation in which exposure to a drug induces changes that result in a diminution of one or more of the drug's effects over time.

Processes of Care

Biomedical

- Basic principles of pain management (Fig. 3.4)
  - Use the least invasive and most readily available and acceptable (to the patient/caregiver) agent/route of administration possible. This is usually the oral route.
  - For continuous pain problems, administer analgesics on a regularly scheduled basis, "around-the-clock" (ATC), rather than on a prn basis. Sustained- or continuous-release formulations make this easier.
  - Treat breakthrough pain.
- **MODERATE OR SEVERE PAIN TREATMENT PROTOCOL**: Analgesic dose titration for pain that is out of control

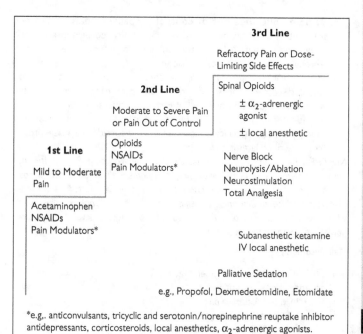

3rd Line

Refractory Pain or Dose-Limiting Side Effects

Spinal Opioids

± α₂-adrenergic agonist

± local anesthetic

Nerve Block
Neurolysis/Ablation
Neurostimulation
Total Analgesia

2nd Line

Moderate to Severe Pain or Pain Out of Control

Opioids
NSAIDs
Pain Modulators*

1st Line

Mild to Moderate Pain

Acetaminophen
NSAIDs
Pain Modulators*

Subanesthetic ketamine
IV local anesthetic

Palliative Sedation

e.g., Propofol, Dexmedetomidine, Etomidate

*e.g,. anticonvulsants, tricyclic and serotonin/norepinephrine reuptake inhibitor antidepressants, corticosteroids, local anesthetics, α₂-adrenergic agonists.

Figure 3.4 Modification of World Health Organization Step Ladder Approach to Pain Control. Reprinted with permission from Fine PG. The evolving and important role of anesthesiology in palliative care. *Anesth Analg* 2005; 100:183–188.

1. Initiate pain treatment protocol within 1 hour for residential/home patients and within 15 minutes for inpatients.
2. Immediately reassess and determine cause of pain.
3. Administer breakthrough pain dose of ordered analgesic; repeat in 15 to 30 minutes if ineffective at bringing pain under control.
4. If pain still poorly controlled, increase breakthrough pain analgesic dose by 50% to 100%.
5. **If pain is well controlled,** increase baseline (ATC) dose of analgesic by 50% and continue with newly adjusted breakthrough pain analgesic.
   a. Reassess in 24 hours and adjust medication dose based on patient's clinical status.
   b. A good rule of thumb is to add total doses of opioid used in previous 24 hours and then consolidate the prn doses into scheduled doses that add up to the 24-hour total. The prn doses can be recalibrated to be approximately 10% of the total daily dose or whatever prn dose is known to sufficiently control the pain.
   c. Adjust bowel regimen accordingly.

6. **If pain continues out of control** (by patient report of pain out of control or behavior suggestive of uncontrolled pain in non–self-reporting patient) 4 hours after initiating protocol, repeat steps 1 through 4 and notify on-call physician.

7. If no significant improvement in pain control 8 hours after initiating protocol, discuss with physician and consider pain management consultation or change to a higher level of care (e.g., general inpatient).

8. If patient is in imminent dying phase and pain is clearly out of control, notify physician of clinical circumstances, and consider ketamine protocol (described later in this section).

NOTE: Establish procedure for frequent reassessment of pain. Pain is often dynamic, persistent, and highly distressing in patients with far-advanced disease states, especially in far-advanced cancer, prior to death. Therefore, frequent reassessment is critical to determine the efficacy of therapy and make readjustments when needed. Successful palliative care and hospice teams develop daily workflows that automate reassessment.

Pharmacotherapy

1. NSAIDs and acetaminophen (Table 3.2)
    a. Indications/advantages
        - Mild to moderate pain
        - Inflammatory pain syndromes, including bone pain
        - Minimal effect on mental functioning

Table 3.2 Acetaminophen and a Selection of Over-the-Counter and Prescription NSAIDs

Drug	>50-kg Dose	<50-kg Dose
Acetaminophen*†	325–650 mg q4–6hr Maximum 4,000 mg/24 hr	10–15 mg/kg q4hr (oral) Maximum 4,000 mg/24 hr
		15–20 mg/kg q4hr (rectal) Maximum 4,000 mg/24 hr
Aspirin*†	4,000 mg/24 hr (q4–6hr dosing)	10–15 mg/kg q4hr (oral) 15–20 mg/kg q4hr (rectal)
Ibuprofen*†	2,400 mg/24 hr (q6–8hr dosing)	10 mg/kg q6–8hr (oral)
Naproxen*†	1,000 mg/24 hr (q8–12hr dosing)	5 mg/kg q8hr (oral/rectal)
Celecoxib‡§	200 mg/24 hr (q12–24hr dosing)	3 mg/kg/24 hr (max 200 mg)
Ketorolac	30–60 mg IM/IV initially, then 15–30 mg q6hr bolus IV/IM or continuous IV/SQ infusion; SHORT-TERM USE ONLY	

* Commercially available in a liquid form
† Commercially available in a suppository form
‡ Minimal effect on platelet function (preferred to nonselective and acetylating NSAIDs in patients subject to bleeding or thrombocytopenia)
§ Reduced GI adverse effects compared with nonselective NSAIDS with short-term or intermittent use

- Supplement with opioid analgesics for moderate to severe pain
- Available over-the-counter in a variety of forms
- Coxibs (COX-2 selective NSAIDs) do not affect platelet adhesion and so are preferred over nonselective NSAIDs when there is a risk of bleeding or patients have thrombocytopenia. Short-term use is associated with less GI risk.
- No psychological or physical dependence, tolerance, hyperalgesia, or addiction risk

   b. Contraindications/disadvantages
- GI distress and ulceration (nonselective NSAIDs and long-term use of COX-2 selective NSAIDs); minimize risk with use of concomitant proton-pump inhibitor therapy
- Platelet dysfunction/bleeding (nonselective NSAIDs)
- Hypersensitivity reactions (NSAIDs)
- Hepatic/renal impairment (NSAIDs and acetaminophen)
- Risk of cardiovascular and cerebrovascular thrombosis with long-term NSAID use (selective and nonselective)

2. Opioid analgesics (Tables 3.3 and 3.4)

   a. Indications: moderate to severe pain, ineffectively controlled with nonopioid analgesics, or when nonopioids are contraindicated

   b. Contraindications
- Allergy or history of sensitivity or dysphoric reactions
- Agonist-antagonist drugs: pentazocine, butorphanol, nalbuphine
- Meperidine (especially in patients with renal insufficiency and history of seizures)

   c. Precautions: anticipate, prevent, and treat opioid-related bowel dysfunction

Table 3.3 Approximate Equianalgesic Doses of Most Commonly Recommended Opioids Analgesics*

Drug	Parenteral Dose	Enteral Dose
Morphine†	10 mg	30 mg
Codeine	Not recommended	200 mg
Fentanyl‡	50–100 mcg	
Hydrocodone		30 mg
Hydromorphone	1.5 mg	7.5 mg
Levorphanol§	2 mg	4 mg
Methadone§	See Table 3.4	
Oxycodone#		20–30 mg
Oxymorphone**	1 mg	10 mg

* Dose conversion should be closely monitored because incomplete cross-tolerance may occur.

† Available in continuous- and sustained-release formulations lasting 8 to 24 hours

‡ Also available in both transdermal and oral transmucosal forms

§ These drugs have long and variable half-lives so accumulation can occur; close monitoring during first few days of therapy is very important.

Available in several continuous-release doses that last 8 to 12 hours

** Available as immediate- (q4–6hr) and extended-release (q12hr dosing) formulations

Table 3.4 Dosing Guidelines for Oral Methadone

Daily Oral Morphine Dose Equivalents	Conversion Ratio of Oral Morphine to Oral Methadone
<100 mg	3:1 (i.e., 3 mg morphine to 1 mg methadone)
101–300 mg	5:1
301–600 mg	10:1
601–800 mg	12:1
801–1,000 mg	15:1
>1,000 mg	20:1

Due to incomplete cross-tolerance and variable potency, it is recommended that when switching to methadone, the initial dose is 50% to 75% of the equianalgesic dose, but be prepared to provide rescue doses of an immediate-acting short-half-life opioid (e.g., morphine, hydrocodone, oxycodone, hydromorphone, oxymorphone) while achieving steady-state doses of methadone (up to 5 to 7 days of tid dosing).

  d. Dose conversions (opioid rotation): Changing from one opioid to another, or one route to another, requires calculation based upon reference to a standard conversion table, a safety step reduction, and a patient-specific step consideration.
  e. Indications for opioid rotation
    — Occurrence of intolerable adverse effects during dose titration
    — Poor analgesic efficacy despite aggressive dose titration
    — Problematic drug–drug interactions
    — Preferences or need for a different route of administration
    — Change in clinical status (e.g., concern about drug abuse or the development of malabsorption syndrome) or clinical setting that suggests benefit from an opioid with different pharmacokinetic properties
    — Financial or drug-availability considerations
• Guidelines for opioid rotation
  • STEP 1
    — Calculate the equianalgesic dose of the new opioid based on the equianalgesic table.
    — If switching to any opioid other than methadone or fentanyl, identify an "automatic dose reduction window" of 25% to 50% lower than the calculated equianalgesic dose.
      • Select a dose closer to the upper bound (50% reduction) of the reduction if the patient is receiving a relatively high dose of the current opioid regimen, is not Caucasian (based on ethnicity-related studies of drug metabolism), or is elderly or medically frail.
      • Select a dose closer to the lower bound (25% reduction) of the reduction if the patient does not have these characteristics or is undergoing a switch to a different route of systemic drug administration using the same drug.
    — If switching to methadone, identify this window at 75% to 90% lower than the calculated equianalgesic dose. For individuals on very high opioid doses (e.g., 1,000 mg morphine equivalents/day or higher), use great caution in converting to methadone at doses of 100 mg or

greater per day; consider inpatient monitoring, including serial electrocardiographic (EKG) monitoring.

— If switching to transdermal fentanyl (sizes available: 12, 25, 50, 75, and 100 mcg/hr), calculate dose conversions based on the equianalgesic dose ratios stated in the product package insert ("complete prescribing information").

• STEP 2

— Perform a second assessment of pain severity and other medical or psychosocial characteristics to determine whether to apply an additional increase or decrease of 15% to 30% to enhance the likelihood that the initial dose will be effective for pain, or, conversely, unlikely to cause withdrawal or opioid-related side effects.

— Have a strategy to frequently assess initial response and titrate the dose of the new opioid regimen to optimize outcomes.

— If a supplemental "rescue dose" is used for titration, calculate this at 5% to 15% of the total daily opioid dose and administer at an appropriate interval. If an oral transmucosal fentanyl formulation is used as a rescue dose, begin dosing at one of the lower doses irrespective of the baseline opioid dose.

f. Safe storage and disposal: Patients and caregivers should be advised to keep all opioid analgesics and other controlled substances under "lock and key," except for an immediately needed dose of breakthrough pain medication or the next dose of a scheduled medication. Disposal of excess or expired medications is very important in order to prevent accidental usage, especially by children, or diversion. Most tablets, capsules, and liquids should be mixed with dirt or cat litter and placed in usual trash receptacles. Most opioids and other controlled substances should be flushed down the toilet. Opioid patches should be folded over on themselves and flushed down the toilet.

g. Driving and functional safety instructions: There are inadequate data from which to make definitive recommendations from available studies. Each patient's circumstances need to be evaluated on their own merits, including disease-related and drug-related impairments that would make driving or other activities dangerous for the patient or others. At the very least, patients (and their caregivers) should be counseled against driving during dose titration and stabilization of opioids and other CNS-depressant drugs.

h. Opioid analgesics: specific features, caveats, cautions, and quirks

• General Principle: In the setting of liver disease with dysfunction, initial doses of opioids should be reduced, but at normal dosing intervals, when hepatic impairment is mild. As hepatic insufficiency worsens, longer dosing intervals may be necessary.

Morphine

• One of the lowest-cost immediate-release and controlled-release agents due to several generic formulations

• Some patients cannot tolerate morphine due to itching, headache, dysphoria, or other adverse effects.

- The metabolites of morphine (morphine-3-glucuronide and morphine-6-glucuronide) may contribute to sedation, myoclonus, and psychotomimetic effects.
- Common effects such as sedation and nausea often resolve within a few days.
- Convert to an equianalgesic dose of a different opioid if adverse effects exceed benefit.
- Anticipate adverse effects, especially constipation, nausea, and sedation, and prevent or treat appropriately.
- Oral morphine solution can be swallowed, or small volumes (1/4 to 1 ml = 5 to 20 mg) of a proprietarily available concentrated solution (20 mg/ml) can be placed under the tongue, recognizing that most of the effect is obtained by enteral absorption after swallowing.
- Morphine's bitter taste may be prohibitive in unflavored forms. "Immediate-release" tablets are not recommended for patients who cannot swallow.

Fentanyl

- Transdermal fentanyl (fentanyl patch): Opioid-naïve patients should be titrated to effective analgesia using short-acting or "immediate-release" opioid analgesics, and then converted to transdermal fentanyl, based upon conversion tables provided in the product prescribing information. See "opioid rotation" earlier in this topic for conversion from another opioid to transdermal fentanyl or from transdermal fentanyl to another opioid formulation. The lowest dose of transdermal fentanyl is 12 mcg/hr, and this may be suitable for low-weight and frail elderly patients, or as an alternative delivery route in patients on relatively low or intermediate doses of opioids (30 to 60 mg oral morphine equivalents per 24 hours) but who can no longer use oral agents. Time to peak and steady-state blood levels for patients starting the patch is usually 18 to 24 hours. Make sure other rapid-onset dosage forms of an opioid analgesic are available during this time period and for breakthrough pain later on. Although the currently available fentanyl patch is formulated for 72-hour use, end-of-dose failure often occurs as early as 48 hours. Close monitoring of efficacy, duration of effect, breakthrough pain episodes and medication use, and adverse effects is important during the first several days of use and during periods of advancing disease with increasing pain, until a stable pattern of effectiveness is reached.

Instructions to Patients

1. Place patch on the upper body in a clean, dry, hairless area.
2. Check daily to make sure patch is not peeling off or has fallen off. If this is consistently problematic, an occlusive dressing should be applied.
3. Avoid heat application over the patch as this will accelerate absorption of medication into body and poses risk of overdose.
4. Choose a different site when placing a new patch, then remove the old patch.
5. Remove the old patch or patches and fold sticky surfaces together, then flush down the toilet.
6. Wash hands after handling patches.

7. All unused patches (patient discontinued use or deceased) should be removed from wrappers, folded in half with sticky surfaces together, and flushed down the toilet.

- Oral transmucosal fentanyl for cancer breakthrough pain (formulations: lozenge on a stick, buccal patch, buccal tablet, sublingual spray, nasal spray): For adults, start with the lowest dose of the preferred formulation for breakthrough pain, and monitor efficacy, advancing to higher-dose units as needed. Onset of pain relief can usually be expected within 10 to 15 minutes after beginning use. Any remaining partial units should be disposed of safely by following instructions in complete prescribing information; patients and caregivers should be counseled about safe storage and disposal and provided with written information.

Buprenorphine

- Partial mu-agonist available in transdermal patch and buccal film formulations; indicated for patients with severe pain for whom other opioids are ineffective or poorly tolerated, or other delivery routes are not feasible
- Buprenorphine transdermal patch: 5-, 10-, 20-mcg/hr transdermal patch dose strengths
  - Initial dosing: 5-mcg/hr patch applied once weekly; titrate up as necessary, or if previously on opioid (up to 80 mg oral morphine equivalent/day) may start on 5- to 10-mcg/hr patch once weekly (medication for breakthrough pain should also be provided)
  - Dose adjustments: generally recommended after 7 days and not more frequently than after 3 days
  - Doses 40 mcg/hr or higher may be associated with QT prolongation.
  - Buprenorphine patch is worn for 7 days; has a well-defined ceiling effect for respiratory depression and respiratory rate rarely drops below 10 breaths per minute (50% of baseline).
- Buprenorphine buccal film: available in dosage strengths of 75, 150, 300, 450, 600, 750, and 900 mcg
  - For opioid-naïve patients, initiate therapy with 75 mcg once daily or q12hr, as tolerated, for at least 4 days before increasing dose to 150 mcg q12hr.
  - Conversion from other opioids to buprenorphine buccal film: Taper current daily opioid dose to 30 mg oral morphine sulfate equivalents (MSE) or less prior to initiating therapy with buprenorphine buccal film.
  - For patients taking less than 30 mg oral MSE, initiate therapy with 75 mcg once daily or q12hr.
  - For patients taking 30 to 89 mg oral MSE, initiate therapy with 150 mcg buprenorphine buccal film q12hr following analgesic taper.
  - For patients taking 90 to 160 mg oral MSE, initiate therapy with 300 mcg buprenorphine buccal film q12hr following analgesic taper.
  - For patients taking greater than 160 mg oral MSE, consider alternative analgesic.
  - Buprenorphine buccal film doses of 600, 750, and 900 mcg are only for use following titration from lower doses of buprenorphine buccal film.

- Do not abruptly discontinue buprenorphine buccal film in a physically dependent patient.
- For patients with severe hepatic impairment: Reduce the starting and incremental dose by half that of patients with normal liver function.
- For patients with oral mucositis: Reduce the starting and incremental dose by half that of patients without mucositis.

Hydromorphone

- Hydromorphone is five to eight times more potent than morphine, permitting analgesic equivalence at lower doses and smaller volumes.
- Hydromorphone can be administered through PO, parenteral (SQ, IM, IV), PR, or intraspinal (epidural and intrathecal) routes.
- Hydromorphone's relatively short half-life of elimination (2 to 3 hours) facilitates dose titration. Onset of action occurs within 15 minutes after parenteral administration and within 30 minutes after PO or PR administration.
- Since hydromorphone is highly soluble in water (up to a maximum concentration of about 300 mg/ml), it is particularly suitable for SQ administration, including continuous subcutaneous infusion (CSCI) and patient-controlled analgesia (PCA).
- Hydromorphone is hydrophilic and extensively distributes in the cerebral spinal fluid (CSF) on epidural administration.
- A high-potency preparation (10 mg/ml) is commercially available for opioid-tolerant patients. This preparation is particularly useful for CSCI in patients where small volumes are necessary.
- Side effects associated with hydromorphone are qualitatively similar to those associated with opioids in general and most often include constipation, nausea, and sedation. Hydromorphone may be preferred in patients with decreased renal clearance in order to prevent toxic metabolite accumulation associated with high-dose morphine.

Levorphanol and Methadone

- These drugs are useful in selected patients as long-acting analgesics due to their long biological half-lives, making dosing intervals (q6–8hr) relatively convenient. The potential for drug accumulation prior to achievement of steady-state blood levels (four to six doses) puts patients at risk for oversedation and respiratory depression. Close monitoring for excessive sedation is required by an observant caregiver. Recent evidence suggests that even low doses of methadone may put patients at risk for arrhythmias due to prolongation of the QT (repolarization) interval. Caution needs to be exercised in patients with electrolyte abnormalities or cardiac conduction abnormalities, and when escalating doses of the drug. Nonlinear dose equivalency of methadone requires close attention to dosing recommendations and extensive experience.

Oxymorphone

- Oxymorphone is the active metabolite of oxycodone.
- Oral oxymorphone is about three times as potent as oral morphine; that is, in patients whose opioid receptor systems are responsive to both drugs,

an opioid-naïve patient taking 3 mg of oral morphine will obtain the same pain relief from 1 mg of oral oxymorphone.

- In patients with cancer pain, the equianalgesic dose ratio between extended-release oxymorphone and controlled-release oxycodone was 1:2.
- The occurrence of side effects is qualitatively and quantitatively similar for the two drugs at equianalgesic doses.
- Available in immediate-release, extended-release, and rectal suppository formulations

Tramadol

- Centrally acting analgesic
- Binds weakly to the mu-opioid receptor, inhibits the reuptake of serotonin and norepinephrine, and promotes neuronal serotonin release
- The World Health Organization (WHO) places tramadol on step 2 of the ladder as an option for treating mild to moderate cancer pain.
- Maximum daily dose is 400 mg/24 hours; in patients more than 75 years old, maximum dose is 300 mg/24 hours.
- High-quality studies in patients with noncancer neuropathic pain confirm its efficacy in treating these painful conditions.
- Adverse effects resemble those of opioids, and caution is advised when using tramadol with SSRIs, monoamine oxidase inhibitors, or tricyclic antidepressants, given the potential for serotonin syndrome.
- Available in immediate-release form as a single agent and in combination with acetaminophen; also available in an extended-release preparation
- Contraindications include risk of seizures in patients with lowered seizure threshold.

Tapentadol

- Tapentadol is a dual-mechanism analgesic, with both mu-opioid agonist effects and norepinephrine reuptake inhibition that is believed to amplify the analgesic potency. It is indicated for moderate to severe acute and chronic pain in adults. Currently available in "immediate-release" tablets (50-, 75-, 100-mg dosage strengths) and "extended-release" tablets.
- The initial immediate-release dose is 50 to 100 mg q4hr (although a second dose can be given 1 hour after the initial dose), with a maximum dose of 600 mg/24 hours.
- Associated with significantly lower incidences of nausea and/or vomiting and constipation, and a significantly lower rate of treatment discontinuation and withdrawal symptoms compared with oxycodone
- Renally cleared inactive metabolite after glucuronidation, so relatively safer in patients with renal insufficiency than opioids with active metabolites (e.g., morphine). There is no significant interaction with liver microsomal enzymes, so there are minimal drug–drug interactions.

Sustained- or Continuous-Release Enteral Formulations

• Several opioids are now available in sustained- or continuous-release form, facilitating compliance and maintaining blood levels between dosing intervals for improved overall control of continuous types of pain.

• Morphine: Commercially available continuous-release pill formulations of morphine last 8 to 24 hours. The continuous-release formulations have similar effects when administered PR, applied with a small amount of water-based lubricant to ease insertion (no encapsulation is necessary). A sustained-release morphine formulation of pellets in a capsule is available that lasts up to 24 hours but cannot be used PR; the capsules can be opened and the contents sprinkled onto a palatable food (e.g., applesauce) as an alternative to swallowing them whole.

• Oxycodone: Continuous-release oxycodone lasts 8 to 12 hours and is available in several dose sizes, starting at 10 mg.

• Oxymorphone: Continuous-release oxymorphone lasts 12 hours and is available in several dose sizes, starting with 5 mg.

• Tramadol and tapentadol are both available in extended-release formulations; see full prescribing information for dose recommendations.

NOTE: Chewing or crushing continuous-release formulations causes them to be IMMEDIATE RELEASE, potentially subjecting the patient to overdosage.

i. Preventing and Treating Opioid Adverse Effects

• Constipation: Always begin a prophylactic bowel regimen when commencing opioid analgesic therapy:
  • Avoid bulking agents (e.g., psyllium) because these tend to cause a larger, bulkier stool, increasing desiccation time in the large bowel.
  • Encourage fluid (fruit juice) intake.
  • Encourage dietary regimens (use of senna tea and fruits).
  • For pharmacotherapy, refer to previous topic on constipation.
  • For opioid-induced constipation refractory to treatment with above interventions, consider the peripheral opioid antagonist agents methylnaltrexone (subcutaneous injection of 0.15 mg/kg [maximum 12 mg] daily) and naloxegol (12.5 to 25 mg PO daily) (see discussion on constipation earlier in this section).

• Excessive sedation: After dose titration for appropriate pain control, and after other correctable causes have been identified and treated if possible, use of psychostimulants may be beneficial:
  • Dextroamphetamine 2.5 to 5 mg PO every morning and midday
  • Methylphenidate 5 to 10 mg PO every morning and 2.5 to 5 mg midday
  • Adjust both dose and timing to prevent nocturnal insomnia.
  • Monitor for undesirable psychotomimetic effects (agitation, hallucinations, irritability).
  • Modafinil 100 to 200 mg PO every morning. This is a relatively safe and effective CNS stimulant that is well tolerated in most patients, but it is relatively expensive.

• Respiratory depression: This is rarely a clinically significant problem for opioid-tolerant patients in pain. When undesired depressed consciousness occurs along with a respiratory rate below 8/min or hypoxemia (O_2 saturation less than 90%) associated with opioid use, cautious and slow titration of naloxone should be instituted. Excessive administration may cause abrupt opioid reversal with pain and autonomic crisis. Dilute one ampule of naloxone (0.4 mg/ml) 1:10 in injectable saline (final concentration 40 µg/ml) and inject 1 ml every 2 to 3 minutes while closely monitoring level of consciousness and respiratory rate.

- Nausea/vomiting: Common with opioids, but habituation occurs in most cases within several days. Assess for other treatable causes. Doses of antiemetics as follows are initial doses, which can be increased as required:
  - Metoclopramide 10 mg PO/IV q6hr
  - Diphenhydramine 25 mg PO/IV q6hr
  - Prochlorperazine 25 to 50 mg PO/PR q6hr
  - Promethazine 25 to 50 mg PO/PR q6hr
  - Haloperidol 0.5 mg IV q6hr or 2 mg PO q6hr
  - Droperidol 1.25 to 2.5 mg IM or IV q6hr
  - Ondansetron 4 mg PO/IV q8hr
- Myoclonus: Occurs more commonly with high-dose opioid therapy. Use of an alternative drug is recommended, especially if using morphine, due to metabolite accumulation. A lower dose of the substitute drug may be possible due to incomplete cross-tolerance:
  - Clonazepam 0.5 mg PO q6–8hr may be useful in treating myoclonus in patients who are still alert and able to communicate and take oral preparations. Increase as needed and tolerated.
  - Diazepam 2 to 5 mg IV as needed to control myoclonus in imminently dying patients with IV access may be helpful.

NOTE: In patients with neuroendocrine cancers, consider serotonin syndrome when evaluating myoclonus; it may exist in a triad of mental status changes, autonomic hyperactivity (i.e., tachycardia), and neuromuscular symptoms.

- Opioid-induced neurotoxicity: This is a clinical syndrome including delirium, myoclonus, and/or increased generalized pain with neuropathic features (e.g., allodynia) with escalating opioid doses. Treatment may be reduction of the opioid dose, rotation to a dissimilar opioid, and/or supplementation with NMDA receptor modulators (e.g., methadone, ketamine, magnesium).
- Pruritus: Most common with morphine, thought to be due to histamine release, but can occur with most opioids. Treatment-induced sedation must be viewed by the patient as an acceptable tradeoff:
  1. Antihistamines
     - Diphenhydramine 25 to 50 mg PO/IV q6hr
     - Hydroxyzine 25 mg PO q6hr
  2. Benzodiazepines
     - Lorazepam 1 mg SL/PO/IV q6hr
     - Hypogonadism: Chronic opioid use can result in testosterone suppression in men, resulting in hypogonadic symptoms such as lethargy, depression, and decreased libido. Total and free testosterone levels may need to be checked. If testosterone insufficiency is confirmed,

then replacement therapy may be warranted if consistent with goals of care and life expectancy.

    j. Tamper-resistant and abuse-deterrent formulations: Several new formulations of oral opioids are now available that are intended to reduce intentional reformulation (crushing and solubilizing for nasal inhalation [snorting] or injecting [shooting], or smoking). The cost of these newer formulations is greater than conventional formulations, but consideration is warranted in patients who have indications for opioid analgesia but are at high risk of abuse or diversion.

    k. Naloxone for opioid overdose: Most states have now legalized distribution of the opioid antagonist naloxone for use by laypersons and first responders. The FDA has approved two formulations: one for injection via an auto-injector and the other a nasal spray, both available by prescription. For patients who are at high risk of opioid overdose, providing a prescription and instructions/counseling to caregivers may be warranted.

Pain-Modulating Drugs ("Adjuvant Analgesics")

- Basic principle: Always consider the addition of pain-modulating agents when there is a specific pathophysiological indication (e.g., bone pain, neuropathic pain), when there is inadequate pain control with primary analgesic therapy alone, when there is sleep disturbance, or when opioid adverse effects predominate (Tables 3.5 and 3.6).

- Pain crises: The first approach to treating pain that has increased beyond the patient's level of comfort is to methodically evaluate the cause, in order to determine the most therapeutically specific means to treat it, while ensuring comfort as quickly and effectively as possible. Table 3.7 outlines a basic approach to immediate analgesic treatment for patients taking ATC opioid analgesics. The hospice physician and IDT should be notified as soon as possible throughout all phases of treatment to ensure that the most appropriate comprehensive care plan is considered and actualized. The patient's primary care physician and other consulting physicians should be notified in a timely manner, depending on their specifications regarding ongoing communication of patient status.

- Most somatic and visceral pain is controllable with appropriately administered analgesic therapy. Some neuropathic pains (e.g., invasive and compressive neuropathies, plexopathies, and myelopathies) may be poorly responsive to analgesic therapies, short of inducing a deeply sedated state. Widespread bone metastases or end-stage pathological fractures may present similar challenges.

- Differentiate terminal agitation or anxiety from "physically" based pain, if possible. Terminal symptoms unresponsive to rapid upward titration of opioid may respond to benzodiazepines (e.g., diazepam, lorazepam; refer to "Agitation and Anxiety" and "Imminent Death" earlier in this section).

- Make sure drugs are getting absorbed. The only guaranteed route is the IV route. Although this is to be avoided unless necessary, if there is any question about absorption of analgesics, parenteral access should be established.

Table 3.5 Pain-Modulating Drugs

DAILY ADULT STARTING DOSE

Drug	Dose Range	Route(s) of Administration	Indications
Corticosteroids			Cerebral edema, spinal cord compression, bone pain, neuropathic pain
Dexamethasone	2–4 mg initial dosing; titrate to bid, tid or qid as needed	PO/IV/SQ	
Prednisone	15–30 mg tid or qid	PO	
Tricyclic antidepressants	10–25 mg q HS	PO	Neuropathic pain, sleep disturbance
Amitriptyline			
Desipramine			
Imipramine			
Nortriptyline			
Doxepin			
Anticonvulsants	Initial dosing, to be titrated up as needed and tolerated		Neuropathic pain
Clonazepam	0.5–1 mg q HS–bid–tid	PO	
Carbamazepine	100 mg qd–tid	PO	
Gabapentin	100 mg qd–tid	PO	
Pregabalin	25–50 mg qd (titrate to bid or tid dosing)	PO	
Local Anesthetics			Neuropathic pain
Mexiletine	150 mg qd–tid	PO	
Lidocaine	10–25 mg/hr	IV or SQ infusion	
Lidocaine 5% transdermal patch: apply to healthy skin overlying painful areas			
Bisphosphonates (see Table 3.4)			
Calcium channel blockers			
Nifedipine	10 mg tid	PO	Ischemic pain, neuropathic pain, smooth muscle spasms with pain

- Neuropathic pain treatment: Choice of agent(s) should be based on clinical circumstances, potential for problematic adverse effects (e.g., anticholinergic effects from TCAs, life expectancy, cost–benefit analysis). Neuropathic pain commonly requires a nonopioid (adjuvant analgesic) combined with

Table 3.6 Comparison of Commonly Used Parenteral and Oral Bisphosphonates in Cancer Patients With Metastatic Bone Disease

Bisphosphonate Generic Name (Brand Name)	Efficacy in Metastatic Bone Disease	Formulations	Effective Dose
Ibandronate* (Boniva)	Effective by oral and IV routes	IV	6-mg infusion over 1–2 hours q3–4weeks
		Oral (2.5-mg tablet)	50 mg/day
Pamidronate* (Aredia)	Oral route not effective in multiple myeloma or breast cancer; IV route is effective	IV (3-mg/ml, 10-ml vial and 9-mg/ml, 10-ml vial)	90-mg infusion over 2 hours q3–4weeks
Zoledronic acid* (Zometa)	IV route very effective, but no oral preparation available	4 mg/5 ml 5-ml vial	4-mg infusion over 15 minutes q4weeks

* Approved in the United States and recommended by the American Society of Clinical Oncologists (ASCO) for treatment of breast cancer patients and symptomatic bone metastases in men with prostate cancer. Bisphosphonates do not appear to influence disease progression or patient survival; however, they should be considered as a palliative option in advanced disease.

Table 3.7 Analgesic Protocol for Escalating Pain in Opioid-Tolerant Patients

Time (hr)	Treatment
0	Definition of pain out of control: Continuous pain >4 to 5/10 not responsive to current analgesic Rx and distressing to patient 1. Bolus dose (PO, SL, PR, IV, SQ) 50% of equivalent hourly dose with immediate release dose of opioid analgesic and 2. Increase ATC doses 50% (notify physician and rest of IDT as soon as time allows).
1	3. If pain still out of control after 1 hour, re-bolus as per No. 1.
2	4. If no appreciable change, notify physician for further orders.
3 to 4	5. If recommendations by hospice/primary care physician(s) do not lead to adequate pain control (pain continues >4 to 5/10 and distressing to patient): Recommend: 1) Opioid rotation (i.e., equivalent dose of alternative opioid analgesic). 2) Parenteral opioid administration (if not already route of administration) with dose titration at bedside.
6 to 8	6. If pain continues out of control, contact medical director to consider other pain management options. 7. Consider continuous care versus general inpatient care. 8. Review indications for other approaches to pain control.

an opioid for optimal pain control. Adjuvant analgesics for neuropathic pain include:

- Tricyclic antidepressants (nortriptyline, desipramine)
- SNRIs (duloxetine, venlafaxine)
- Calcium channel alpha(2)-delta ligands (gabapentin, pregabalin)
- Sodium channel blockers (intravenous and topical lidocaine)
- Topical capsaicin mexiletine
- N-methyl-d-aspartate receptor antagonists (methadone, ketamine)
- Cannabinoids (tetrahydrocannabinol [THC], cannabidiol [CBD]): There is anecdotal evidence in humans and laboratory research in animals supporting use of the cannabinoids THC and CBD, alone and in various combinations, for the treatment of neuropathic pain. Regulatory issues confound research, availability of pharmaceutical-grade formulations, evidence-based guidance, and federally sanctioned legal use at this time.

Pain Crises

- Severe pain that is poorly responsive to basic approaches to analgesic therapy merits consultation with a pain management consultant as quickly as possible. Radiotherapy, anesthetic, or neuroablative procedures may be indicated.

- Consider spinal/epidural opioid/local anesthetic approaches, neurolytic celiac plexus block, or spinothalamic tractotomy. Expertise in these techniques is required; credentials AND experience should be determined in advance of referral.

- From a case-management standpoint, these interventions can add greatly to quality of life and decrease costs if a patient's pain is inadequately controlled by appropriate dose titration of opioid analgesics and adjuvants.

- Ketamine protocol: For truly intractable end-stage pain, parenteral administration of ketamine will provide relief for the patient and ease the great distress that witnessing such agony can cause family and other caregivers who need or want to remain in attendance.

  - Bolus: Ketamine 0.1 mg/kg IV. Repeat as often as indicated by the patient's response. Double the dose if no clinical improvement in 5 to 10 minutes. Follow the bolus with an infusion. Decrease opioid dose by 50%.

  - Infusion: Start ketamine at 0.015 mg/kg/min IV (about 1 mg/min for a 70-kg individual). SQ infusion is possible if IV access is not attainable. In this case, use an initial IM bolus dose of 0.3 to 0.5 mg/kg. Decrease opioid dose by 50%.

  - It is advisable to administer a benzodiazepine (e.g., diazepam or lorazepam) concurrently to mitigate against the possibility of hallucinations or frightening dreams, since patients under these circumstances may never be able to communicate such experiences.

  - Observe for problematic increases in secretions; treat with glycopyrrolate, scopolamine, or atropine (see "Imminent Death" topic on secretions).

  - Dexmedetomidine, an alpha-2 agonist, provides an alternative to ketamine therapy, especially when deep sedation is desired. Use of this agent requires blood pressure and airway monitoring. Dosing: 1 µg/kg over 10 minutes followed by 0.6 µg/kg/hr.

Breakthrough Pain

• This is very common in patients with chronic pain and is defined as intermittent episodes of moderate or greater pain that occurs despite control of baseline continuous pain (Fig. 3.5).

• Although best studied in cancer patients, there is evidence that patients with other pain-producing, life-limiting diseases experience breakthrough pain a few times a day, lasting moments to many minutes. The risk of increasing the ATC analgesic dose is increasing adverse effects, especially sedation, once the more short-lived, episodic breakthrough pain has remitted.

1. Subtypes and treatment
   a. Incident pain: Pain that is predictably elicited by specific activities. Use a rapid-onset, short-duration analgesic formulation in anticipation of pain-eliciting activities or events. Adjust dose to severity of anticipated pain or the intensity/duration of the pain-producing event. Past experience will serve as the best guide.
      • Conventionally, oral morphine solution or other immediate-release oral formulations of opioid analgesics have been used most commonly, in order to avoid parenteral administration, but relatively long and inconstant/unpredictable onset times coupled

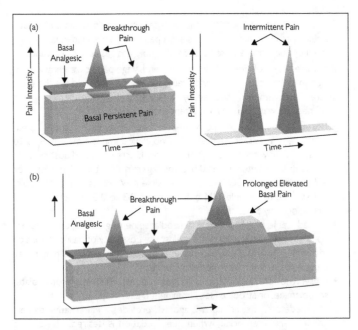

Figure 3.5 (a) Differentiating breakthrough pain from intermittent pain.
(b) Differentiating breakthrough pain from prolonged elevated basal pain.

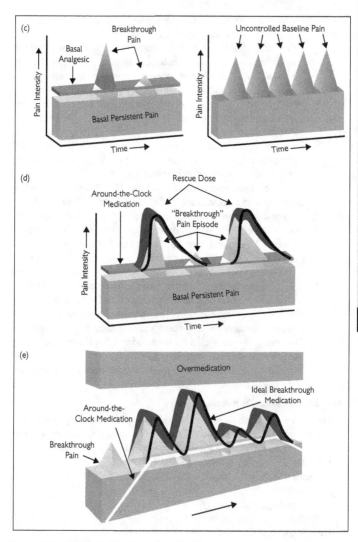

Figure 3.5 (*Continued*) (c) Differentiating breakthrough pain from uncontrolled baseline pain. (d) The rescue dose as a conceptual foundation for breakthrough pain. (e) Management of baseline and breakthrough pain. Adapted with permission from Fine PG. *The Diagnosis and Treatment of Breakthrough Pain*. New York: Oxford University Press, 2008.

with duration of effect exceeding the typical breakthrough pain episode limit the utility of this traditional approach.

- Oral and nasal transmucosal fentanyl (proprietary approved formulations: lozenge on a stick, buccal tablet, buccal patch, SL spray, nasal spray) is an effective, noninvasive means of treating these symptoms in opioid-tolerant patients. IV bolus dosing for patients with IV access may be necessary in those circumstances where oral or transmucosal drugs cannot be used (PCA devices may be helpful).

b. Spontaneous pain: Unpredictable pain, not temporally associated with any activity or event. These pains are more challenging to control. Use of adjuvants for neuropathic pains may help diminish the frequency and severity of these types of pains (see Table 3.5). Otherwise, immediate treatment with a potent, rapid-onset opioid analgesic is indicated.

c. "End-of-dose failure" is the phrase used to describe pain that occurs toward the end of the usual dosing interval of a regularly scheduled analgesic. This results from declining blood levels of the ATC analgesic prior to administration or uptake of the next scheduled dose. Appropriate questioning will ensure rapid diagnosis of end-of-dose failure. Shortening the dose interval to match the onset of this type of breakthrough pain should remedy this problem. For instance, a patient who is taking continuous-release morphine q12hr whose pain "breaks through" after about 8 to 10 hours is experiencing end-of-dose failure. The dosing interval should be increased to q8hr. If the dose interval becomes too short to make compliance easy, then it is reasonable to increase the dose by 25% to 50%, monitoring closely for therapeutic and adverse effects.

Nonpharmacological Treatments

- There is robust academic and community-based interest in complementary and alternative medicine (CAM) therapies in treating pain as part of a comprehensive and integrative approach to pain care. These include:
  - Heating and cooling techniques
  - Electrical stimulation (e.g., TENS)
  - Ultrasound
  - Massage (e.g., Reiki therapy)
  - Mindfulness meditation
  - Music therapy
  - Aromatherapy
  - Herbal therapies
  - Cognitive-behavioral therapies (CBT)
  - Yoga therapies (including specific breathing techniques)
- The decision to use one or more of these approaches is a function of the IDT's expertise and experience; access to trained and "credentialed" volunteers; and patient/family expectations, values, interests, and goals. Although risks are low, it is important to ensure patient safety with regard

to physical modalities (heat, ice, electricity, positioning, allergies/sensitivities, and potential drug–herbal interactions).

Interventional Treatments for Cancer Pain

- While the use of conventional analgesics (opioids and NSAIDs) and adjuvants for cancer pain remains a mainstay in accordance with the traditional WHO analgesic ladder, this approach does not produce adequate pain control in an estimated 20% to 30% of patients (see Fig. 3.4). As advanced illness and end-of-life care evolve, and as we gain more sophisticated and patient- and condition-specific approaches to treating pain, hospice and palliative care professionals will need to team up with pain medicine experts in order to optimize pain treatment for their patients. The pain-related variables that need to be assessed at the outset and throughout the course of an IDT's care of a patient, in order to determine when and how urgently to call in an interventional pain specialist, include:
  - Conditions that lend themselves to definitive pain relief by neural blockade (e.g., pancreatic cancer)
  - Life expectancy of the patient (days, weeks, months)
  - Degree of distress experienced by the patient and family due to poorly controlled pain
  - Goals and priorities of the patient (comfort, physical function, alertness)
  - Adverse effects of conventional analgesics (nausea/vomiting, sedation, cognitive impairment, bowel dysfunction)
  - Access to and expertise/experience of a consultant interventional pain specialist
  - Opportunity costs (home-based vs. facility-based treatment; physical/emotional burden of transport; availability of transport; financial burden)
- Traditionally, hospice patients have not had access to interventional pain treatment, largely due to concerns about costs due to constraints of hospice funding streams. However, IDTs should have the expertise to analyze the cost-effectiveness of all treatment options, including all opportunity costs—especially those associated with delays in obtaining adequate pain control from conventional analgesic therapies, adverse effects of conventional analgesics therapies (especially high-dose opioids), and staff time involved in responding to poorly controlled pain. Early and repeated pain assessments and ongoing analyses of overall effectiveness of treatment should be done in order to ensure timely, safe, and effective pain treatment in all cases.
- The most common procedures that the IDT should consider in those patients who are not responding favorably to noninvasive pain control approaches include vertebral augmentation, local anesthetic and/or neurolytic injections, and intrathecal drug delivery.

Vertebral Augmentation

- Metastatic cancer is the most common hospice diagnosis associated with severe pain. Spine lesions are particularly common in patients with multiple myeloma as well as breast, prostate, renal cell, thyroid, and lung cancers. Vertebral body lesions may lead to vertebral compression fractures that can cause debilitating pain and reduced function.

- While some patients improve with rest, analgesics, physical therapy, and bracing, pain can persist or be so severe that it compromises function, sleep, and social interactions, leading to extreme suffering. Open surgical repair carries the risk of significant morbidity and is reserved for existing or impending myelopathy in patients with a protracted life expectancy.

- Vertebroplasty and kyphoplasty are minimally invasive procedures used to treat painful vertebral compression fractures. Vertebroplasty aims to stabilize painful fractures with injection of the bone cement polymethyl methacrylate into the vertebral body. Kyphoplasty differs in that the injection of cement is preceded by the inflation of a percutaneously placed intravertebral balloon to create a cavity, with or without attempted restoration of vertebral height. The most recent data preferentially support the use of kyphoplasty in the cancer population.

- Neural blockade (see Table 3.8)

- Intrathecal therapy (see Table 3.9)

- Palliative radiation therapy: Radiation therapy also has an important place in the treatment of pain, and similar to close association with a pain medicine specialist, IDTs should have consultancy relationships established with radiation therapists (see Appendix 1).

Table 3.8 Indications and Injection Procedures for Commonly Encountered Cancer-Related Pain Conditions

Procedure Location	Indications	Possible Adverse Effects
Celiac Plexus	Upper abdominal visceral pain from malignant tumors of the pancreas, hepatobiliary system, small intestine, stomach, spleen, ascending colon, or adrenal glands	Transient hypotension Diarrhea Transient or permanent spinal cord damage (rare)
Superior Hypogastric Plexus	Visceral pelvic pain from malignant primary or metastatic tumor in the ovary, uterus, cervix, bladder, rectum, or prostate	Neuraxial injection Discitis Bladder injury Intravascular injection Retroperitoneal hematoma
Ganglion of Impar	Perineal pain from rectal or anal cancers or metastatic perineal lesions	Rectal perforation Local infection Local bleeding Intravascular injection

Table 3.9 Common Indications and Medications Used for Commonly Encountered Cancer-Related Pain Conditions

Drug	Mechanism	Indications	Adverse Effects	Notes
Morphine	Mu-agonist	First-line therapy for nociceptive or mixed pain, second-line therapy for neuropathic pain	Sedation, nausea, pruritus, respiratory depression, urinary retention	FDA-approved for intrathecal delivery
Hydromorphone				
Fentanyl				Typically added as 2nd opioid or after failure of initial opioid
Sufentanil				
Ziconotide (Prialt)	N-type calcium channel blockade	First-line or second-line therapy for nociceptive and neuropathic pain	Mood disturbance, visual hallucinations, ataxia, elevated creatine kinase	FDA-approved for intrathecal delivery
Bupivacaine	Sodium channel blockade	First-line therapy for neuropathic pain, second-line therapy for nociceptive pain	Motor weakness, urinary retention, hypotension, bradycardia	Typically used in combination with an opioid
Clonidine	Alpha-2 agonist	Third-line therapy for nociceptive or neuropathic pain	Ataxia, sedation, bradycardia, postural hypotension	Serious withdrawal syndrome with abrupt discontinuation
Baclofen	Central-acting GABA-agonist	Third-line therapy for nociceptive or neuropathic pain, especially if spasticity is present	Motor weakness, bradycardia, hypotension	Potentially fatal withdrawal syndrome with abrupt discontinuation

Goals/Outcomes

- Pain out of control (patient self-report of more than 3/10 pain, or pain greater than patient's acceptable level) is brought under control within 48 hours of admission to hospice
- Pain out of control is assessed and responded to with effective intervention within predetermined time frames in all patients so that no patient dies with pain out of control
- Analgesic adverse effects and side effects are prevented or effectively managed in all patients

Documentation in the Medical Record

Initial Assessment

- Findings from comprehensive pain assessment are organized in a standard format according to putative diagnosis, mechanism(s), contributing factors, functional limitations and patient goals/values.
- Current pain management regimen
- Patient/caregiver understanding/expectations/goals of pain management
- Concerns regarding opioids
- Review of systems pertinent to analgesic use: bowels, balance, memory, etc.
- Counseling regarding driving or other dangerous activities

Interdisciplinary Progress Notes

- Ongoing findings from pain reassessment
- Baseline pain scores
  - Breakthrough pain frequency and severity
  - Effects on function, sleep, activity, social interaction, mood, etc.
- Types and effects (outcomes) of interventions, including adverse effects
- Bowel function, sedation, nausea/vomiting assessments
- Documentation of specific instructions, patient/caregiver understanding, compliance
- Patient/caregiver coping

IDT Care Plan

- Specific pharmacological and nonpharmacological interventions to be performed by which members of the IDT
- Contingency plans and crisis prevention/intervention plans reviewed as indicated

Recommended Reading

American Pain Society. Definitions related to the use of opioids for the treatment of pain. 2001. Available at http://www.ampainsoc.org/advocacy/opioids2.htm.

Chou R, Fanciullo GJ, Fine PG, et al. Clinical guidelines for the use of chronic opioid therapy in chronic noncancer pain. *J Pain* 2009; 10(2):113–130.

Christo PJ, Mazloomdoost D. Cancer pain and analgesia. *Ann NY Acad Sci* 2008; 1138:278–298.

Ferrell B, Fine PG, Herr K, et al., for the AGS Panel on Persistent Pain in Older Persons. Clinical guideline for the pharmacological management of persistent pain in older persons. *J Am Geriatrics Soc* 2009; 57:1331–1346.

Fine PG, Mahajan G, McPherson ML. Long-acting and short-acting opioids: appropriate use in chronic pain management. *Pain Med* 2009; 10(S2):S1–10.

Fine PG, Finnegan T, Portenoy RK. Protect your patients, protect your practice: practical risk assessment in the structuring of opioid therapy in chronic pain. *J Fam Pract* 2010; 59(9, Suppl 2):S1–S16/

Fine PG, Portenoy RK. Establishing "best practices" for opioid rotation: conclusions of an expert panel. *J Pain Symptom Management* 2009; 38(3):418–425.

Knotkova H, Fine PG, Portenoy RK. Opioid rotation: the science and limitations of the equianalgesic dose table. *J Pain Symptom Management* 2009; 38(3):426–439.

O'Connor AB, Dworkin RH. Treatment of neuropathic pain: an overview of recent guidelines. *Am J Med* 2009; 122(10 Suppl):S22–32.

Pergolizzi J, Aloisi AM, Dahan A, et al. Current knowledge of buprenorphine and its unique pharmacological profile. *Pain Pract* 2010; 10(5):428–450.

Pergolizzi J, Böger RH, Budd K, et al. Opioids and the management of chronic severe pain in the elderly: consensus statement of an international expert panel. *Pain Practice* 2008; 8(4):287–313.

Sindt J, Brogan S. Interventional treatments of cancer pain. In: Ashburn MA, Fine PG, eds. *Pain Management* (Anesthesiology Clinics). Philadelphia: Elsevier Health Sciences, 2016.

Subramaniam K, Subramaniam B, Steinbrook R. Ketamine as an adjuvant analgesic to opioids: a quantitative and qualitative review. *Anesthesia Analgesia* 2004; 99:482–495.

Webster LR, Fine PG. Approaches to improve pain relief while minimizing opioid abuse liability. *J Pain* 2010; 11:612–620.

Pruritus

SITUATION: Chronic or recurrent itching that has a negative impact on the patient's physical or emotional well-being

Causes

• Overly dry skin (xerosis) and moist skin (maceration) are common and easily treated causes.

• Contact dermatitis, drug reactions (allergy), fungal infection, and skin infestations should be considered and either ruled out or treated.

• Cholestasis or hepatobiliary disorders are common occurrences in many advanced disease states, due to drug reactions, accumulation of bile salts, or obstruction.

• Hodgkin's disease, gastric carcinoid, and cutaneous infiltration in malignant diseases cause pruritus.

- The majority of patients experiencing chronic renal failure will have this symptom, with up to 60% of dialysis patients experiencing uremic pruritus.
- Diabetic pruritus without any associated skin findings occurs in 3% of diabetic patients.
- Pruritus frequently accompanies the use of intrathecally or epidurally administered opioids, with a reported incidence between 30% and 100%.

Findings

- Self-report of itching or behavior suggestive of pruritus in noncommunicative patient (e.g., scratching, restlessness)
- Excoriated skin from excessive scratching
- Skin rash (with or without signs of systemic disease such as conjunctival pallor or icterus, lymphadenopathy, thyromegaly, splenomegaly, or hepatic disease)
- Scratching without relief of symptoms
- Fitful sleep
- Mood alteration (irritability)

Assessment

- The key to treatment of pruritus (sensation of itching) is identification of the cause; inadequate treatment can lead to excoriation and secondary infection, sleep deprivation, mood alteration (irritability), and generalized discomfort.
- History of symptoms as revealed by patient or observant caregiver, paying particular attention to the temporal nature of the symptoms, location, and exacerbating and alleviating factors
- Identification of likely disease-related causes
- Physical examination of the skin
- Identification of environment-related causes

Processes of Care

- For xerosis or macerated skin, use lubricating or drying techniques and materials, respectively; moisturizers and/or occlusive dressings are recommended after washing and drying.
- Nonspecific pharmacotherapy can be used until specific treatments take effect or as an adjunct if adequate resolution does not occur:
  1. Sedating agents with some antihistamine activity (H1 antagonist), especially at night, will promote rest and sleep. Titrate choice of drug slowly and monitor therapeutic effects versus undesirable side effects:
     a. Hydroxyzine (25 to 50 mg PO q6hr)
     b. Doxepin (10 to 50 mg PO q HS)
     c. Promethazine (25 to 50 mg IV q4–6hr)
     d. Diphenhydramine (25 to 50 PO/IV q6hr)

e. Cyproheptadine (pediatrics: 0.25 mg/kg/day; adults: 0.5 mg/kg/day maximum dose) starting with a low dose and titrating upward, bid or tid PO dosing (syrup = 2 mg/tsp; tablets = 4 mg/tab)

2. Serotonin reuptake inhibitor therapy, such as paroxetine 10 to 30 mg PO qd, has been demonstrated to be effective in palliating pruritus not caused by cholestasis or primary dermatologic disease.

3. Gabapentin may be beneficial in patients with uremic, idiopathic, and brachioradial pruritus.

4. Cholestatic pruritus that is not amenable to drug changes or stenting may respond to salt-binding drugs, such as cholestyramine (4 g PO qid), but this drug is generally not well tolerated in very ill individuals. Rifampin 300 to 600 mg/day and opioid antagonists such as IV naloxone and oral naltrexone have been of benefit for patients not able to tolerate cholestyramine in cholestatic pruritus. Additional palliative medications include:
   a. Maalox 15 ml PO q6hr
   b. Methyltestosterone 25 mg SL bid (caution in hormone-sensitive tumors, except in end-stage symptom control)
   c. Ondansetron 4 to 8 mg (IV/PO) q8–12hr

5. Capsaicin cream or patch is anecdotally reported as being effective, although its use may be limited by abnormal or irritated skin at the site of symptoms.

6. Skin infiltration by malignancies, such as breast cancer, might respond to NSAID therapy, if tolerated. Use maximum anti-inflammatory doses (e.g., naproxen 15 to 20 mg/kg/day in divided doses; ibuprofen 30 to 40 mg/kg/day in divided doses)

7. Opioid-induced pruritus is usually short-lived, with patients becoming rapidly habituated to this effect. Changing to an equally potent dose of another drug (especially a synthetic derivative, because histamine release is common with morphine-like compounds) is one alternative. Use of nonspecific pharmacotherapy as suggested above will generally attenuate symptoms during the habituation phase. Patients with spinal opioid-delivery systems may benefit from low-dose naloxone infusion (1 µg/kg/hr) or oral naltrexone (12.5 mg PO daily), slowly increasing the dose as needed.

8. Suspected skin infestation (e.g., scabies) or fungal infection should be treated with the appropriate primary therapy, complemented by nonspecific palliative therapies, as above, to treat symptoms until the cause is effectively treated. Inflammatory skin disorders may respond to topical corticosteroid therapy (e.g., hydrocortisone 0.5% to 1% or triamcinolone acetonide 0.025% cream).

Goals/Outcomes

- Relief of physical and emotional distress associated with pruritus
- Prevention of skin breakdown and infection
- Improved sleep

Documentation in the Medical Record

Initial Assessment

- Severity, location(s), and duration/timing of symptoms
- Aggravating and alleviating factors
- Etiology of symptoms

Physical Examination Findings

- Effects on sleep, mood, social interactions, activities
- Skin appearance, lesions, rashes, scratch-marks/excoriation

Interdisciplinary Progress Notes

- Effects of interventions, including possible adverse drug reactions

IDT Care Plan

- Specific interventions and follow-up plans

Recommended Reading

Etter L, Myers SA. Pruritus in systemic disease; mechanisms and management. *Dermatol Clin* 2002; 20:459.

Gunal AI, Ozalp G, Yoldas TK, et al. Gabapentin therapy for pruritus in hemodialysis patients: a randomized, placebo-controlled, double-blind trial. *Nephrol Dial Transplant* 2004; 19:3137.

Lysy J, Sistiery-Ittah M, Israelit Y, et al. Topical capsaicin—a novel and effective treatment for idiopathic intractable pruritus ani: a randomised, placebo controlled, crossover study. *Gut* 2003; 52(9):1323–1326.

Phan NQ, Bernhard JD, Luger TA, Stander S. Antipruritic treatment with systemic mu opioid receptor antagonist: a review. *J Am Acad Dermatol* 2010; 63:680.

Tandon P, Rowe BH, Vandermeer B, Bain VG. The efficacy and safety of bile acid binding agents, opioid antagonists, or rifampin in the treatment of cholestasis-associated pruritus. *Am J Gastroenterol* 2007; 102:1528.

Xander C, Meerpohl JJ, Galandi, et al. Pharmacological interventions for pruritus in adult palliative care patients. *Cochrane Database Syst Rev* 2013; 9(6):CD008320.

Seizures

SITUATION: Patient/caregiver distress and potential morbidity from uncontrolled seizure

Seizures are frightening to caregivers and exhausting for patients. In addition, they create risk of injury. They should be prevented if at all possible, and a plan for immediate treatment should be in place for those patients who are susceptible. These include patients with a preexisting seizure disorder and those with brain tumors or brain metastases.

Causes

- Preexisting seizure disorder
- Structural brain abnormality

- Primary cerebral neoplasm
- Metastatic disease to the brain
- Prior stroke
- Metabolic disorders
  - Hypomagnesemia
  - Hypocalcemia
  - Hyponatremia
  - Hypoglycemia/hyperglycemia
  - Hypoxia/anoxia
  - Uremia
  - Liver failure
- Infection
- Drug abstinence syndromes (e.g., alcohol, benzodiazepines, barbiturates, baclofen)
- New use or increased dosage of medications that lower seizure threshold in at-risk patients (e.g., phenothiazines such as prochlorperazine, chlorpromazine; butyrophenones such as haloperidol, droperidol; tricyclic antidepressants such as amitriptyline, doxepin, nortriptyline, desipramine)

Findings

- Physical manifestation of seizure varies depending on area and amount of brain involved.
- Possible manifestations include:
  - Frank convulsive motor activity (generalized seizure)
  - Tonic motor posturing (generalized seizure)
  - Focal motor convulsion (limited to one side, or one body part) (partial seizure)
  - Forced eye deviation to one side (partial or generalized seizure)
  - Altered mental status in at-risk patient (complex partial seizure)
- Associated findings may include:
  - Altered mental status associated with disseminated cancer
  - Headache, nausea, spontaneous projectile vomiting associated with increased intracranial pressure
  - "Aura" as a prodrome to seizure activity (e.g., visual, auditory, or olfactory sensory change)
  - Period of altered physical or mental function with gradual return to baseline after generalized seizure

Assessment

- Review of past medical history should reveal seizure disorder.
- In patients who have had seizures, determine seizure risk: frequency of events, date of most recent event, characteristics of each seizure, prior use of antiepileptic medications.
- Differentiate seizures from other mimics, such as muscle twitching (myoclonic jerks) and alterations in level of consciousness due to nonseizure causes.

- If already on seizure prophylactic medications, review schedule, dose, and adverse effects/toxicity/drug–drug interactions.
- If "breakthrough" seizure activity while on medication, may want to check blood levels or empirically alter medication regimen per physician consultation
- Determine most appropriate level of care based on patient's seizure history/risk and current care setting.

Processes of Care

Psychosocial/Practical

- Educate patient/caregiver as to importance of prophylactic therapy and acute seizure management.
- Assess caregiver's previous experience, understanding, and preparedness for seizure management.
- Protect patient from falling and from sharp or hard surfaces.
- Do not actively restrain the patient or try to put anything in the mouth; turn the patient onto a side and lift the chin to help maintain the airway and minimize aspiration risk if possible.
- Reorient patient slowly and calmly. Do not give anything to eat or drink until full recovery of sensorium.

Biomedical

- Correct readily treatable metabolic or systemic disturbances (electrolytes, glucose, urinary tract infection, fever).
- Reevaluate medication list for any medications that decrease seizure threshold, as listed above.
- Consider pharmacological management: choice based on available route of administration, medication interactions, coexisting hepatic or renal disease, and cost.
- Pharmacological management (see Tables 3.10 and 3.11)
  - Acute treatment
    a. Assess patient safety as above (turn on side, move sharp objects away).
    b. Note seizure characteristics and duration.
       - Self-limited seizure—supportive care, await return to baseline. Reassess prophylactic regimen and assess for metabolic disarray, infection, and fever.

Table 3.10 Partial List of Commonly Used Anticonvulsants

Medication	Routes Available	Metabolism	Interactions	Cost
Phenytoin	PO, IV	Hepatic, inducing	Many	Low
Valproic acid	PO, IV, PR	Hepatic, inhibiting	Many	Low
Levetiracetam	PO, IV	Renal	Few	Moderate
Phenobarbital	PO, IV, PR, SQ	Hepatic, inducing	Many	Very low
Carbamazepine	PO, PR	Hepatic, inducing	Many	Low

Table 3.11 Dosing of Commonly Used Antiepileptic Drugs

Generic Drug	Brand name	Usual daily Dose
Carbamazepine	Tegretol	600–2,000 mg/day in three or four doses/day
Carbamazepine Controlled release	Tegretol XR	600–2,000 mg/day in two doses/day
Gabapentin	Neurontin	1,800–3,600 mg/day in three doses/day
Lamotrigine	Lamictal	100–400 mg/day in one or two doses/day
Levetiracetam	Keppra	1,000–3,000 mg/day in two doses/day
Phenobarbital	Luminal	30–180 mg/day in two doses/day
Phenytoin	Dilantin	150–500 mg/day in one or two doses/day
Topiramate	Topamax	200–400 mg/day in two doses/day
Sodium valproate Divalproex sodium	Depakene Depakote	400–2,000 in one or two doses/day

- Ongoing or frequent seizure with no return to baseline in between—initial management with benzodiazepine followed by other agents if necessary. Assess for metabolic disarray, infection, and fever, and treat if possible and appropriate as related to the patient's goals of care

c. Benzodiazepine choice for acute treatment typically is based on available route of administration. During ongoing seizure, avoid oral route if possible due to secretions, aspiration risk, and caregiver safety (Table 3.12).

d. For refractory seizures that do not cease with benzodiazepine administration

- IV access: Give phenytoin IV infusion 20 mg/kg over 20 to 30 minutes in normal saline solution; an additional 5 to 10 mg/kg can be given if seizures persist.
- IV or SQ access, or refractory to phenytoin administration: Infuse phenobarbital 20 mg/kg IV at a rate of 100 mg/min.

Table 3.12 Benzodiazepine Choice for Acute Treatment

Route Available	Medication	Dose
IV	Lorazepam	0.1 mg/kg (typically divided in two or three doses)
PR	Diazepam	0.2–0.5 mg/kg (typically started as 5–10 mg PR and repeated as needed)
SQ	Midazolam	0.2 mg/kg followed by 0.05–0.2 mg/kg/hr

e. In patients with known cerebral tumor or metastases, adjuvant treatment with dexamethasone to decrease cerebral edema may be beneficial (1 mg/hr IV/SQ infusion).

- Drug management of the dying patient with seizure disorder at home if continuation of antiepileptic drug is considered necessary
  - If on valproate: As swallowing decreases, suspension or oral sprinkles can be used. When patient becomes unable to take PO, switch to rectal preparation, with no dose adjustment.
  - If on carbamazepine: As swallowing decreases, switch to suspension. When patient becomes unable to take PO, administer by suppository, with no dose adjustment.
  - If on phenobarbital: Switch to parenteral solution administered rectally or give by suppository.
  - If on levetiracetam: can try to give suspension rectally; may need to double the dose

Goals/Outcomes

- Prevention of seizures
- Preparedness of caregiver in the event of seizure activity
- Prevention of seizure-related potential morbidity/injury

Documentation in the Medical Record

Initial Assessment

- History of seizures, seizure control regimen, and effectiveness
- Current disease process likely to pose seizure risk
- Level of understanding/preparedness of patient/caregiver regarding seizures and seizure prevention/control

Interdisciplinary Progress Notes

- Incidence and types of seizure activity
- Patient/caregiver instruction
- Understanding and adherence to seizure prevention plan
- Seizure prophylaxis toxicities/adverse effects
- Reassessment of appropriateness of level of care

IDT Care Plan

- Seizure precautions and prevention/treatment plan and interventions defined
- Follow-up and contingency plans

Recommended Reading

Andersohn F, Schade R, Willich SN, Garbe E. Use of antiepileptic drugs in epilepsy and the risk of self-harm or suicidal behavior. *Neurology* 2010; 75(4):335–340.

Epilepsy Foundation. First aid for seizures. Available at http://www.epilepsyfoundation.org/about/firstaid/index.cfm (accessed January 2016).

Epilepsy Foundation. Prolonged or serial seizures (status epilepticus). Available at http://www.epilepsyfoundation.org/about/types/types/statusepilepticus.cfm (accessed January 2016).

Krouwer H, Pallagi J, Graves N. Management of seizures in brain tumor patients at the end of life. *J Palliat Med* 2000; 3:465–475.

National Institute of Neurological Disorders and Stroke. Seizures and epilepsy: Hope through research. Available at http://www.ninds.nih.gov/disorders/epilepsy/detail_epilepsy.htm (accessed January 2016).

Tradounsky G. Seizures in palliative care. *Can Fam Physician* 2013; 59:951–955.

Skeletal Muscle and Bladder Spasms

SITUATION: Pain and associated distress from spontaneous or incident-related muscle spasms or cramps involving skeletal muscles or bladder

Causes

- Primary neuromuscular diseases
- Spinal cord or plexus injury
- Neuromuscular effects of tumor compression/infiltration
- Immobility
- Metabolic disturbances (electrolyte abnormalities)
- Infection
- Bladder distention
- Indwelling urinary catheter

Findings

- "Charlie horse" of calf, thigh, low back, intercostal, neck muscles most common
- Sense of urinary urgency or crampy, colicky pain in lower pelvis; may also occur during or after voiding
- Bladder pain syndrome manifests as bladder pain, frequency, nocturia, and urgency.

Assessment

- Elicit patient history of bladder or skeletal muscle spasms causing pain during review of systems and physical examination.
- Evaluate timing of muscle spasms in relation to activity, time of day or night, position. Muscle spasm will create nociceptive impulses from the muscle to the CNS; increases in pain lead to increases in spasm (pain–spasm–pain cycle).
- Check for dysuria, urinary frequency, feeling of fullness even after voiding, inability to initiate urinary stream.
- Consider benefits/burdens of electrolyte or urine evaluation based on probabilities of etiology and impact of results on treatment plan.

Processes of Care

• Direct primary therapy at cause if feasible and not overly burdensome.

Skeletal Muscle Spasms

• Nonpharmacological interventions
  1. Help patient reposition frequently if prone to cramps/spasms; use pillows, bolsters for support and bed rails, trapeze if patient has strength to reposition self.
  2. Passively and slowly stretch/elongate cramping muscles with continuous steady force until contraction discontinues.
  3. Gently massage with lotion.
  4. Actively warm body parts with warm moist towel.

• Pharmacological management
  • Skeletal muscle relaxants are divided into two categories:
    1. Antispastic (for conditions such as cerebral palsy and multiple sclerosis)
       NOTE: Antispastic agents (e.g., baclofen, dantrolene) should not be prescribed for musculoskeletal conditions because there is sparse evidence to support their use and there are serious adverse effects whose potential risks must be weighed against benefits.
       a. Benzodiazepines: Titrate carefully and balance therapeutic effects against sedation and potential memory impairment.
          i. Diazepam 2 to 10 mg PO/IV titrated to effect. Repeat based on duration of response.
          ii. Alternatively, lorazepam 1 to 5 mg liquid concentrate can be used in patients where the PO or SL route is preferred.
          iii. Alternatively, clonazepam 0.5 to 2.0 mg PO may be preferable in patients with concurrent neuropathic pain due to its purported pain-relieving actions.
       b. Baclofen 5 to 10 mg PO up to tid, based on response and adverse effects (sedation, urinary retention, generalized weakness)
    2. Antispasmodic agents (for musculoskeletal conditions); the choice of a skeletal muscle relaxant should be based on its adverse effect profile, tolerability, and cost (Table 3.13).
       a. First-line therapy for typical back pain syndromes (e.g., low back strain): acetaminophen and NSAIDs
       b. Second-line therapy: cyclobenzaprine or tizanidine; the sedative properties of tizanidine and cyclobenzaprine may benefit patients with insomnia caused by severe muscle spasms
       c. Metaxalone and methocarbamol may be useful in patients who cannot tolerate the sedative properties of cyclobenzaprine or tizanidine; methocarbamol costs substantially less than metaxalone.
    3. Quinine sulfate tablets (one or two) PO q HS as tolerated (GI intolerance may be dose-limiting) have been reported to be useful in idiopathic muscle cramping (especially nocturnal cramps).
    4. Ongoing trials of cannabis extracts (THC/CBD) in MS patients with muscle spasms have demonstrated some benefit, with approval in

Table 3.13 Skeletal Muscle Relaxants (Antispasmodic Agents)

Drug Generic (Brand)	Recommended Dosage (PO)	Most Common Adverse Effects	Comments	Monthly cost ($)*
Carisoprodol (Soma)	350 mg qid; not recommended for children younger than 12 years	Dizziness, drowsiness, headache; rare idiosyncratic reactions (mental status changes, transient quadriplegia, and temporary loss of vision) after first dose; allergy-type reactions may occur after the first to fourth dose; may be mild (e.g., cutaneous rash) or more severe (e.g., asthma attack, angioneurotic edema, hypotension, or anaphylactic shock); antihistamines, epinephrine, or corticosteroids may be needed	Physical or psychological dependence may occur; withdrawal symptoms may occur with discontinuation; possible respiratory depression when combined with benzodiazepines, barbiturates, opioids, or other muscle relaxants; contraindicated in acute intermittent porphyria; FDA pregnancy category C	72–100 (generic), 590 (brand)
Chlorzoxazone (Parafon Forte)	Adults: 250–750 mg tid or qid Children: 125–500 mg tid or qid; or 20 mg/kg daily in three or four divided doses	Dizziness, drowsiness, red or orange urine, GI irritation and rare GI bleeding; hepatotoxicity (rare); discontinue with elevated liver function test	Avoid use in patients with hepatic impairment; possible respiratory depression when combined with benzodiazepines, barbiturates, opioids, or other muscle relaxants; FDA pregnancy category C	15–77 (generic), 180 (brand)

SECTION 3 Clinical Processes and Symptom Management

Table 3.13 Continued

Drug Generic (Brand)	Recommended Dosage (PO)	Most Common Adverse Effects	Comments	Monthly cost ($)*
Cyclobenzaprine (Flexeril)	5 mg tid; may increase to 10 mg tid	Anticholinergic effect (drowsiness, dry mouth, urinary retention, increased intraocular pressure); rare but serious adverse effects are arrhythmias, seizures, myocardial infarction	Most-studied skeletal muscle relaxant; long elimination half-life; 5-mg dose as effective as 10-mg dose, with fewer adverse effects; avoid in older patients and in patients with glaucoma; possible drug interaction with CYP450 inhibitors; seizures reported with concomitant use of tramadol (Ultram), so combination should be avoided in patients with medical conditions that may induce seizures; contraindicated in patients with arrhythmias, recent myocardial infarction, or congestive heart failure; FDA pregnancy category B	120–140, (generic) 157 (brand)
Diazepam (Valium)	Adults: 2–10 mg tid or qid Children: 0.12–0.80 mg/kg daily in three or four divided doses	Dizziness, drowsiness, confusion; abuse potential	Also an antispastic agent; long elimination half-life; avoid in older patients and in patients with hepatic impairment; possible drug interaction with CYP450 inhibitors; avoid especially in the first trimester pregnancy category D; FDA	11–23 (generic), 184 (brand)
Metaxalone (Skelaxin)	800 mg tid or qid; not recommended in children younger than 12 years	Drowsiness, dizziness, headache, nervousness; leukopenia or hemolytic anemia (rare); liver function test elevation (rare); nausea, vomiting, and diarrhea (rare); paradoxical muscle cramps	Use with caution in patients with liver failure; possible respiratory depression when combined with benzodiazepines, barbiturates, opioids, or other muscle relaxants; less dizziness and drowsiness than other skeletal muscle relaxants; FDA pregnancy category C	275; generic not available

Drug	Dosage	Side Effects	Comments	Cost*
Methocarbamol (Robaxin)	1,500 mg qid for first 2–3 days, followed by 750 mg qid	Black, brown, or green urine possible; mental status impairment; possible exacerbation of myasthenia gravis symptoms	Possible respiratory depression when combined with benzodiazepines, barbiturates, opioids, or other muscle relaxants; FDA pregnancy category C; reports of fetal abnormalities	15–58 (generic), 176 (brand)
Orphenadrine (Norflex)	100 mg bid; combination products are dosed tid or qid	Anticholinergic effect (drowsiness, dry mouth, urinary retention, increased intraocular pressure); GI irritation, confusion, tachycardia, aplastic anemia (rare); hypersensitivity reaction (with high doses)	Long elimination half-life; reduce dosages in older patients; avoid in patients with glaucoma, cardiospasm, or myasthenia gravis; FDA pregnancy category C	110–140 (generic), 162 (brand)
Tizanidine (Zanaflex)	4 mg initially; may increase by 2–4 mg q6–8hr until relief; do not exceed 36 mg daily	Dose-related hypotension, sedation, and dry mouth; hepatotoxicity—monitor liver function tests at baseline and at 1, 3, and 6 months; withdrawal and rebound hypertension may occur in patients discontinuing therapy after receiving high doses for long period of time; tapering is recommended	Also antispastic agent; do not use with CYP1A2 inhibitors, ciprofloxacin (Cipro) or fluvoxamine (Luvox CR); caution with CNS depressants or alcohol; decreased effectiveness with oral contraceptives; FDA pregnancy category C	329 (generic), 437 (brand)

Note: The table contains only selected highlights about these medications. All of these drugs may cause increased drowsiness with CNS depressants. Caution is advised when prescribing skeletal muscle relaxants in older patients.

CYP, cytochrome P; FDA, U.S. Food and Drug Administration; GI, gastrointestinal.

* For the recommended adult dosage. Estimated cost to the pharmacist based on average wholesale prices (rounded to the nearest dollar) in Red Book (Montvale, NJ: Medical Economics Data, 2007).

27 countries (including Canada and the UK), but not yet the United States.

- Intractable spasms may occasionally require special techniques (e.g., nerve blocks) to manage; consult with a qualified and experienced expert if symptoms do not abate or treatment-related adverse effects are overly burdensome.

Bladder Spasms

- Nonpharmacological management
  - Urinary catheterization
    - To relieve a urinary tract obstruction that can't be otherwise managed for a patient with neurogenic bladder dysfunction, hydronephrosis, and urinary retention that can't be relieved by other definitive means, such as with clean intermittent catheterization
    - To manage urinary incontinence in a patient with a Stage III or IV pressure ulcer and to provide comfort care in terminally ill patients
- Pharmacological management
  1. Antibiotic therapy for infection (per culture and sensitivities, or empirical use of trimethoprim-sulfa or ciprofloxacin)
  2. Phenazopyridine 100 to 200 mg PO QID (caution about staining from pigmented urine)
  3. Oxybutynin 2.5 to 5 mg PO q8–12hr prn (caution about anticholinergic effects)
  4. Belladonna and opium suppositories 16.2 to 30 mg or 16.2 to 60 mg PR q12h prn
  5. Lidocaine irrigation in catheterized patients: add 10 ml of 2% lidocaine to 50 ml saline irrigant, infuse and clamp catheter for 20 to 30 minutes, and then unclamp; useful for short-term relief (less than 2 weeks)
  6. Amitriptyline may be beneficial in persons who can achieve a daily dose of 50 mg or greater in newly diagnosed patients with interstitial cystitis/painful bladder syndrome.
  7. Triple therapy with gabapentin, amitriptyline, and NSAIDs for bladder pain syndrome

Goals/Outcomes

- Eliminate muscle and bladder spasms whenever possible.
- Enable patient/caregiver to be able to palliate muscle spasms quickly and effectively.

Documentation in the Medical Record

Initial Assessment

- Frequency, intensity, location, aggravating/inciting and alleviating characteristics and associated signs and symptoms

Physical Examination Findings

- Likely etiology

Interdisciplinary Progress Notes

- Types of interventions and effects of therapies

• Instruction in prevention and treatment regimens and specific interventions
• Follow-up plan and contingencies

Recommended Reading

Foster HE Jr., Hanno PM, Nickel JC, et al. Effect of amitriptyline on symptoms in treatment-naïve patients with interstitial cystitis/painful bladder syndrome. *J Urol* 2010; 183(5):1853–1858.

Landy S, Altman CA, Xie F. Time to recovery in patients with acute painful musculoskeletal conditions treated with extended-release or immediate-release cyclobenzaprine. *Adv Ther* 2011; 28(4):295–303.

Lee JW, Han DY, Jeong HJ. Bladder pain syndrome treated with triple therapy with gabapentin, amitriptyline, and a nonsteroidal anti-inflammatory drug. *Int Neurourol J* 2010; 14(4):256–260.

Leussink VI, Husseini L, Warnke C, et al. Symptomatic therapy in multiple sclerosis: the role of cannabinoids in treating spasticity. *Ther Adv Neurol Disord* 2012; 5(5):255–266.

Nickel JC, Moldwin R, Lee S, et al. Intravesical alkalinized lidocaine (PSD597) offers sustained relief from symptoms of interstitial cystitis and painful bladder syndrome. *BJU Int* 2008; 103:910.

See S, Ginzburg R. Choosing a skeletal muscle relaxant. *Am Family Physician* 2008; 78(3):365–370.

Weil AJ, Ruoff GE, Nalamachu S, et al. Efficacy and tolerability of cyclobenzaprine extended release for acute muscle spasm: a pooled analysis. *Postgrad Med* 2010; 122(4):158–169.

Witenko C, Moorman-Li R, Motycka C, et al. Considerations for the appropriate use of skeletal muscle relaxants for the management of acute low back pain. *Pharmacy and Therapeutics* 2014; 39(6):427–435.

Skin Breakdown: Prevention and Treatment

SITUATION: Actual or potential skin breakdown leading to patient morbidity and caregiver burden

Causes

• Pressure ulcers resulting from decreased mobility, sensory loss, or impaired mental capacity (decubiti)
• Body fluids causing skin irritation/maceration (incontinence, ostomy sites, wound drainage, etc.)
• Itching/pruritus leading to skin excoriation
• Vascular insufficiency leading to ischemia or stasis ulcers
• Tumor erosion or infiltration
• Poor nutritional status, low albumin level (less than 3.5 mg/dl)
• Friction, abrasion from skin contact surfaces

Findings

- Reddened, irritated skin
- Sources of body fluid/wound seepage
- Nonblanching erythematous skin over pressure areas/bony prominences (e.g., sacrum, hips)
- Partial- or full-thickness ulcers, eschar formation
- Areas of skin excoriation
- Patient may or may not communicate pain.
- Putrid odor from infected wounds

Assessment

- Elicit patient report of painful, irritating, or itchy areas.
- Physical examination of all pressure-bearing areas, especially dorsal surfaces of bedridden and immobile patients, on a daily basis: sacral and coccygeal, greater trochanter, ischial tuberosity, lateral malleolus, heel
- Check for capillary filling over erythematous and blanching skin surfaces.
- Identify source(s) of bodily fluids: sweats, urine, fecal material.
- Determine cause of itching/pruritus (see "Pruritus" above in this section).
- Consider superinfection of open sores/wounds/ulcers by virtue of purulence and odor.
- Assess abrasiveness of skin contact surfaces (e.g., bedclothes, rails, wheelchair, Hoyer lifts).
- Pressure ulcer stages by National Pressure Ulcer Advisory Panel:
  - Stage 1: Nonblanchable erythema of intact skin; the heralding lesion of skin ulceration; darkly pigmented skin may not have visible blanching; its color may differ from the surrounding area
  - Stage 2: Partial-thickness skin loss presenting as a shallow open ulcer with a red–pink wound bed, without slough; may also present as an intact or open/ruptured serum-filled blister
  - Stage 3: Full-thickness skin loss involving damage or necrosis of subcutaneous tissue that may extend down to, but not through, underlying fascia; the ulcer presents clinically as a deep crater with or without undermining of adjacent tissue
  - Stage 4: Full-thickness skin loss with extensive destruction, tissue necrosis, or damage to muscle, bone, or supporting structures (e.g., tendon or joint capsule); slough or eschar may be present on some parts of the wound bed; often undermining and tunneling
  - Unstageable: full-thickness tissue loss with base of the ulcer covered by slough and/or eschar
  - Suspected deep tissue injury: purple/maroon/discolored intact skin or blood-filled blister from damage of underlying soft tissue due to pressure and/or shear; deep tissue injury may be difficult to detect in patients with dark skin. Undermining and tunneling should be measured and documented.
- Assess and identify severity or degree of progressive/additive risk factors, including:

- General physical condition (good, fair, poor, very bad)
- Mental condition (alert, apathetic, confused, stupor)
- Activity (ambulatory, walks with assistance, chair-bound, bed-bound)
- Mobility (full, slightly limited, very limited, immobile)
- Incontinence (none, occasional, frequent urinary incontinence, doubly incontinent)
- Nutritional status (excellent, adequate, inadequate, very poor)
- Sensory responsiveness (painful [rate intensity]; normal sensation or slightly limited, very limited, absent)
- Wound assessment scales can be used to help predict occurrence of pressure ulcers and can be used in conjunction with clinical assessment:
  - Norton scale
  - Braden scale for predicting pressure

Processes of Care

Practical and Biomedical

Prevention

Caregiver education in the following areas will greatly reduce the risk of skin breakdown and the development of pressure ulcers in at-risk patients (see Tables 3.14 and 3.15 and http://www.guideline.gov/search/search.aspx?term=pressure+ulcers):

Table 3.14 Control of Causative and Contributing Factors

Causative and Contributing Factors	Interventions
Infection	Prevention by using clean technique
	Treatment of infection by the use of topical and/or oral antibiotics
Excessive moisture	Prevention by keeping patient clean/dry (moisture barrier creams, diapers, pads, changing linens, etc.), and consider Foley catheter insertion if appropriate, especially when patient is incontinent; aggressively identify and alleviate any causes of excessive moistures
Shear and friction	Prevention by using draw sheets (not "scooting or dragging" patient across sheets), eliminating wrinkles and crumbs in linens, keeping patient from sliding in bed; quickly identifying and eliminating factors creating shear or friction
Altered nutritional status	Prevention by identifying those at risk with nutritional assessment and taking appropriate action as indicated by assessment; encourage patient to eat/drink if this is consistent with patient goal; provide excellent mouth care as well
Unrelieved pressure	Frequent turning/repositioning, pressure relief devices such as overlay, APP mattress; sheepskin and egg-crate mattresses are comfort measures and do NOT relieve pressure; assess bony prominences frequently for signs of redness, blanching, blisters; take immediate action; do not massage area

Table 3.15 Pressure Ulcer Treatment Recommendations

Stage 1	Stage 2	Stage 3 & 4	Unstageable
For pressure points and buttocks *Barrier ointment/cream (daily)*	For infected wounds *Silver antimicrobial (every 1–7 days)*	For infected wounds *Silver antimicrobial (every 1–7 days)*	Stable eschar serves as biological cover and should NOT be removed.
For high-friction areas *Transparent dressings (every 1–7 days)*	No exudate *Transparent dressing (every 1–7 days)* Mild exudate *Hydrogel sheet (every 2–5 days)* Moderate exudate *Hydrocolloid dressing (every 2–7 days)* Severe exudate *Foam dressing (every 1–7 days)*	For cavity that needs to be filled With no to mild exudate *Hydrogel-impregnated gauze (every 1–3 days)* Moderate exudate *Alginate dressing (every 2–4 days)* Severe exudate *Foam dressing (every 1–7 days)*	
		For undermining and tunneling *Alginate dressing foam (every 1–4 days)*	
		For cavity with necrotic tissue *Super-absorbent polymer pad (daily)*	

1. All at-risk individuals should have a systematic skin inspection at least once a day by caregiver(s), paying particular attention to the bony prominences.
2. Skin should be cleansed at the time of soiling and at routine intervals, avoiding hot water, using minimal application of friction, and using mild cleansing agents that minimize irritation and dryness of the skin.
3. Use topical agents (e.g., zinc oxide preparations) that act as barriers to moisture and underpads/briefs that rapidly absorb moisture and present a quick-drying surface to the skin.
4. Avoid massage over bony prominences. Current evidence suggests that this may be harmful.
5. Minimize environmental factors leading to skin drying, such as low humidity and exposure to cold; dry skin should be treated with moisturizers.
6. Skin injury due to friction and shear forces should be minimized through proper positioning, transferring, and turning techniques. Use lubricants, protective films and dressings (e.g., hydrocolloids), and protective padding.

7. At-risk patients should be repositioned at least every 2 hours if this is consistent with established goals/preferences.
8. Apply positioning devices (e.g., pillows, foam pads) to bony prominences (e.g., knees, ankles, heels) to prevent direct contact with each other or hard surfaces.
9. Avoid positioning immobile patients with full weight on trochanter (when in lateral position).
10. Avoid uninterrupted sitting in chair/wheelchair by immobile patients if unable to shift weight from pressure points at least hourly. Balance this risk with overall patient goals/preferences.
11. Do not use donut-type devices in chairs as it causes venous congestion and edema and increases pressure area.
12. A recliner chair's ability to prevent pressure ulcers is still not known.
13. Premedicate patients 30 minutes prior to a large position change for patients with significant pain.

Treatment

1. Repositioning: constant repositioning at least every 2 hours, or every 4 hours if frequent repositioning is too painful or not tolerable
2. Support surfaces (in order of most effective and also most expensive to least effective)
   a. Air fluidized
   b. Low air loss
   c. Alternating air
   d. Static flotation (air or water)
   e. Foam
   f. Standard mattress

NOTE: The appropriate choice of support surface depends on risk factors, presence and severity of ulcers, ability of caregivers to prevent and treat ulcers, and financial resources. Regardless of the chosen support surface to be used, REPOSITIONING is the more important factor in preventing and treating pressure ulcers. Support surfaces that have developed "bottoming out" phenomenon should be replaced.

3. Débridement: The method of ulcer débridement chosen should be based on the patient's condition and individual goals/preferences:
   a. Noninfected ulcers should be débrided using dressings (i.e., hydrocolloids, hydrogels, transparent films, alginates, foams) that maintain moisture within the wound bed, supporting the body's own ability to cleanse itself and allowing enzymes present in wound fluids to break down necrotic tissues.
   b. Enzymatic débridement is accomplished by applying topical débridement agents to devitalized tissue on the wound surface.
   c. The simplest mechanical débridement techniques include hydrotherapy and wound irrigation. Safe and effective irrigation pressures range from 4 to 15 pounds per square inch (psi); the least expensive and most effective devices that deliver pressures within this range are:
      • 60-ml piston irrigation syringe with catheter tip (4.2 psi)
      • 250-ml saline squeeze bottle with irrigation cap (4.5 psi)

- Waterpik at lowest (#1) setting (6.0 psi)
- 35-ml syringe with 19-gauge needle or angiocatheter (8.0 psi)

d. Sharp débridement is rarely indicated except in patients with a relatively long life expectancy and extensive devitalized tissue with infection. Surgical consultation may be required, and pain control should be the highest priority.

e. Myiasis: Effects of using sterile maggots have yet to be determined.

f. Medical-grade honey (*Leptospermum scoparium*) can be used to promote autolytic débridement via high sugar levels; it helps rapidly reduce odor and create a moist wound healing environment when paired with an occlusive, absorbent dressing.

g. Heel ulcers with dry eschar are an exception and need not be débrided if there is no edema, erythema, fluctuance, or drainage. Assess these wounds daily, keeping heels slightly elevated and "floated."

4. Wound cleansing and dressings: Healing/prevention of infection is more likely if fastidious wound cleansing is carried out and appropriate dressings are applied. Active cleansing needs to be balanced against inciting pain and aggravating wound trauma. Routine cleansing should be accomplished with minimal chemical or mechanical irritation/trauma:

a. Cleanse wounds with normal saline; do not use antiseptics.

b. Dress ulcers in a manner that keeps the ulcer bed moist and surrounding skin dry.

c. There are no specific outcomes differences for different choices of moist wound dressings, so select one that is most convenient and least costly, such as film and hydrocolloid dressings.

d. Use antibiotic therapy only if fastidious wound care has otherwise failed to control bacterial colonization (exudate and odor persisting after several days of routine wound care).

- Topical antibiotic trial: silver sulfadiazine or triple antibiotic, monitoring for sensitivity reactions or other adverse effects (also see "Bleeding, Oozing, and Malodorous Lesions")
- **No** topical antiseptics (i.e., povidone–iodine, iodophor, sodium hypochlorite, hydrogen peroxide, acetic acid)
- Charcoal dressings may help reduce odor.
- When used topically, metronidazole gel or crushed tablets applied daily on wounds can eradicate the anaerobes that cause odor.

e. Use appropriate body substance control techniques.

f. Treat pain as indicated in the discussion on "Pain" earlier in this section.

- Aerosolized 0.5% bupivacaine or a paste of aluminum hydroxide–magnesium hydroxide may reduce the need for, or dose of, systemic analgesics.

g. For unstageable ulcers, cover with dry nonsterile dressing.

Goals/Outcomes

- Prevent pressure ulcers
- Limit extent of existing wound (see Table 3.16)

Table 3.16 Determining Appropriate Goals

Protocol	Patient Characteristics	Goal of Wound Care
H	Serum albumin >3.0 and/or patient eating well; no weight loss in past 6 months; patient ambulatory	Healing*
M	Serum albumin 2.8–3.0 and/or fair nutrition; ≤10% weight loss past 6 months; patient somewhat ambulatory but primarily sedentary; peripheral vascular disease and/or diabetic neuropathy	Maintenance†
C	Serum albumin <2.8; poor nutrition; >10% weight loss; primarily or totally bed-bound or chair-bound; peripheral vascular disease and/or diabetic neuropathy	Comfort‡

* Healing: complete healing of wound is expected.
† Maintenance: wound will not become infected or worsen, but not expected to heal.
‡ Comfort: wound will not become infected, may become worse, but patient will be pain-free.

Table 3.17 Protocol H (Goal: Healing)

Problem	Interventions
Wound (describe)	See earlier Treatment section.
	Assess wound for signs/symptoms of infection, treat any infection with adjunctive antibiotics.
	Manage causative and contributing factors, including unrelieved pressure, shear and friction, excessive moisture, altered nutrition.
	Dietary consult as determined by nutritional assessment and IDT
	Pain relief, if needed
	If no evidence of healing within 2 weeks after treatment initiated, reevaluate whether healing is a valid goal by assessing causative factors, nutrition, infection, vascular insufficiency; redefine goal as indicated.
	If goal remains healing, reassess goal and discuss at IDT at least every 2 weeks.

Table 3.18 Protocol M (Goal: Maintenance)

Problem	Interventions
Wound (describe)	See earlier Treatment section.
	Dietary consult as determined by nutritional assessment and IDT
	Pain relief, if needed
	If evidence of worsening of wound, evaluate whether maintenance is a valid goal by assessing causative factors, nutrition, infection, vascular insufficiency; redefine goal as indicated; if goal remains maintenance, reassess goal and discuss at IDT at least every 2 weeks.

Table 3.19 Protocol C (Goal: Comfort)	
Problem	**Interventions**
Wound (describe)	See earlier Treatment section 3: Skin Breakdown: Prevention and Treatment.
	Pain relief, if needed
	Control odor.
	If goal remains comfort, reassess goal and discuss at IDT at least every 2 weeks.

- Eliminate and limit impact and adverse effects associated with skin breakdown if it occurs
- Minimize morbidity and added caregiver burden by constant encouragement, education, teaching, and demonstration of proper skin care protocols

Documentation in the Medical Record

Initial Assessment
- Findings from skin examination (Table 3.17)
- Risk factors for pressure ulcers and skin breakdown
- Patient/family's goals of wound care
- Needs assessment (i.e., support services, caregiver capabilities)

Physical Examination Findings
- Precise location, size and description of lesions.

Interdisciplinary Progress Notes
- Interventions and instructions given
- Results of interventions and ongoing reassessments

IDT Care Plan
- Specific interventions and instructions to caregiver(s) (Table 3.18)
- Follow-up plans and contingencies (Table 3.19)

Recommended Reading

Bolton LL, Girolami S, Corbett L, van Rijswijk L. The Association for the Advancement of Wound Care (AAWC) venous and pressure ulcer guidelines. *Ostomy Wound Manage* 2014; 60(11):24–66.

Eisenberger A, Zeleznik. Care planning for pressure ulcers in hospice: the team effect. *J. Palliat Support Care* 2004; 2(3):283–289.

Kalinski C, Schnepf M. Effectiveness of a topical formulation containing metronidazole for wound odor and exudates control. *Wounds* 2005; 17(4):74–79.

Karopchinsky JA. Pressure ulcers. *MedSurg Nurs* 2015; 24(3):183–184.

Nenna M. Pressure ulcers at the end of life. An overview for home care and hospice clinicians. *Home Healthcare Nurse* 2011; 29(6):350–365.

Zacur H, Kirsner R. Debridement: rationale and therapeutic options. *Wounds* 2002; 14(7 Suppl E.):2E–7E.

Urinary Problems

SITUATION: Urinary retention or incontinence leading to patient distress or increased caregiver burden

Causes

- Benign prostatic hypertrophy (BPH)
- Prostatic malignancy
- Prostatitis
- Bladder atony
- Urinary tract infection
- Medication-induced retention from anticholinergic drugs (e.g., tricyclic anti-depressants) and sympathomimetic drugs
- Fecal impaction with secondary obstruction
- Kinked, blocked, clogged, obstructed urinary (Foley) catheter
- Patient inability to attend to toileting
- Cauda equina syndrome or other spinal/sacral plexus impairment
- Diuretic effect (especially at night)
- Stroke or other CNS impairment

Findings

- Patient or caregiver report of dribbling or frank incontinence
- Urinary urgency, frequency, dysuria
- Small, frequent voids
- Infrequent voiding with "overflow" incontinence
- Bladder spasms
- Palpable bladder on physical examination
- Change in normal urine color/odor/clarity (e.g., dark, bloody, malodorous)

Assessment

- Systems review with patient, if communicative, or caregiver, including abdominal pain, distention, cramps, bowel movements, change in urinary frequency, volume, color, odor, pain while voiding, etc.
- Review medications (especially diuretics, anticholinergics).
- Assess amount and timing of fluid intake.
- Abdominal, pelvic, perineal, genital, rectal examination as indicated by presenting symptoms/signs
- Grossly examine urine (volume, color, odor).

Processes of Care

Practical

- Try to regulate late fluid intake and keep the timing of diuretics to the morning to avoid nocturnal bladder filling.
- Instruct patient/caregiver to have patient void in upright (sitting) position and try to initiate voiding on a fixed schedule to "train" the bladder (i.e., q4hr during the day).

Biomedical

- Adjust anticholinergic medications if at all possible, balancing relative benefits and burdens of therapies, side effects, and "competing" symptom complexes.
- Treat urinary tract infection and bladder spasms as per "Skeletal Muscle and Bladder Spasms" earlier in this section.
- Trial of alpha-1-adrenergic antagonist monotherapy (e.g., terazosin or doxazocin)
- Consider condom catheter (men) or external pouch catheter (men or women) for incontinence, if no evidence of obstruction.
- Teach caregiver care and maintenance of condom catheter system and importance of genital skin care.
- For urinary obstruction or bothersome urinary incontinence, insert urinary catheter (Foley) following aseptic technique.
- Monitor initial urine output: if greater than 1,000 ml, clamp catheter for 15 minutes, and then continue gravity drainage, clamping the catheter for 15 minutes for every additional 500 ml of output
- Irrigate urinary catheters with sterile water on a regular basis; discontinue if no fluid return, and consult physician.
- Consult with physician if unable to pass a standard urinary catheter with minimal effort.
- Instruct caregiver in care and maintenance of indwelling urinary catheter and drainage system (cleansing urinary meatus, observing for obstruction and signs of infection/inflammation around urethral opening/meatus, emptying drainage reservoir, keeping reservoir below level of the patient's bladder).
- Lidocaine 2% ointment or 4% K-Y Jelly may help decrease pain, burning, stinging, and irritation at catheter insertion site.
- Manually disimpact and initiate bowel protocol per discussion in "Constipation" as needed.
- If obstruction is related to an infection and the infection is treated, patient should have a voiding trial.

Goals/Outcomes

- Prevent bladder distention
- Prevent pain or additional morbidity from urinary retention or incontinence

- Minimize distress, additional morbidity, social isolation, and caregiver burden due to incontinence
- If urinary retention or incontinence is an ongoing problem despite treatment, discuss goals of care with the patient and/or caregiver. If in line with the patient's wishes, then refer for further evaluation from a urologist.

Documentation in the Medical Record

Initial Assessment
- Review of urinary symptoms, voiding patterns, fluid intake, medications

Physical Examination Findings
- Effect of urinary problems on caregiver, patient self-image, and social interactions
- Effect of urinary problems on environment (odor, etc.)
- Likely cause(s) of urinary problems

Interdisciplinary Progress Notes
- Specific interventions and results
- Patient/caregiver coping

IDT Care Plan
- Etiology-specific interventions and contingencies with follow-up plan
- Plan for patient/caregiver instruction as required by circumstances

SITUATION: Gross hematuria (visible blood in urine) and/or outflow obstruction from clots, leading to patient/caregiver distress

Causes

- Urinary tract infection
- Prostate cancer (men), bladder or renal cancer (men and women)
- Nephrolithiasis (kidney stones)
- Benign prostatic hypertrophy (men)
- Prostatitis (men)
- Benign essential hematuria
- Pseudo-hematuria (non–hematuria-related reddish urine): myoglobinuria, hemoglobinuria, porphyria, bilirubinuria, drugs (phenothiazines, rifampin, pyridium), foods (beets, rhubarb)
- Trauma
- Adverse effect of anticoagulation

Findings

- Patient or caregiver report of blood in urine or red-colored urine
- Blood and/or blood clots in urine or bladder catheter
- Decreased urine output

- Increased bladder/urethral pain
- Bladder spasms

Assessment

- Evaluate urine for gross hematuria: as little as 1 ml of blood may change hue of urine.
- Review medical history, medications (anticoagulants [consider benefit vs. burden of checking bleeding time], drugs causing pseudo-hematuria), dietary intake.
- Systems review with patient, if communicative, or caregiver, including abdominal pain, distention, cramps, bowel movements, change in urinary frequency, volume, color, odor, pain while voiding, etc.
- If in line with patient's goals of care, consider urinalysis and urine culture.
- Abdominal, pelvic, perineal, genital, rectal examination as indicated by presenting symptoms/signs; if history indicates, evaluate for outflow tract obstruction (physical exam for palpable bladder, ultrasound bladder scan)

Processes of Care

- Review goals of care.
- If in line with goals of care, and negligible amount of gross hematuria (i.e., not interfering with normal urine flow, no physical distress), reassure patient and caregivers.
- If indicated, treat urinary tract infection and bladder spasms as per "Skeletal Muscle and Bladder Spasms" earlier in this section.
- If gross hematuria with clots, consider inserting urinary catheter (Foley) following aseptic technique (see above for insertion technique). Monitor urine output, and provide standard indwelling catheter management.
- Consult with physician if unable to pass a standard urinary catheter with minimal effort; patient may require Coudé (bent-tip) catheter for easier insertion. If still unable to pass catheter, patient may require suprapubic catheter placement by urologist.
- Consult with physician if gross hematuria or blood clots persist; patient may require larger-bore double-lumen catheter (20 to 24 Fr) for easier drainage, or a three-way catheter for intermittent or constant bladder irrigation.
- Always continue optimal symptom management for physical discomfort/distress related to etiology and management of gross hematuria.

Goals/Outcomes

- Prevent bladder distention, enable adequate urine outflow
- Minimize distress, additional morbidity, social isolation, and caregiver burden due to gross hematuria
- If hematuria is an ongoing problem despite treatment, discuss with the patient and/or caregiver about goals of care. If in line with the patient's wishes, then refer for further evaluation from an urologist.

Documentation in the Medical Record

Initial Assessment

- Review of urinary symptoms, voiding patterns, fluid intake, medications

Physical Examination Findings

- Effect of urinary problems on caregiver, patient self-image, and social interactions
- Effect of urinary problems on environment (incontinence, blood loss, etc.)
- Likely cause(s) of gross hematuria

Interdisciplinary Progress Notes

- Specific interventions and results
- Patient/caregiver coping

IDT Care Plan

- Review of patient's goals of care related to complications of gross hematuria and management strategies
- Etiology-specific interventions and contingencies with follow-up plan
- Plan for patient/caregiver instruction as required by specific circumstances, including when to contact hospice case manager

Recommended Reading

Barrisford GW, et al. Acute urinary retention. http://www.uptodate.com/contents/acute-urinary-retention (accessed August 12, 2015).

Feldman A, et al. Etiology and evaluation of hematuria in adults.http://www.uptodate.com/contents/etiology-and-evaluation-of-hematuria-in-adults (accessed August 12, 2015).

Mercadante S, Ferrera P, Casuccio A. Prevalence of opioid-related dysuria in patients with advanced cancer having pain. *Am J Palliat Care* 2011; 28(1):27–30.

Xerostomia (Dry Mouth)

SITUATION: Dry oral mucous membranes, lips, palate, throat, and tongue, often attended by cracking/bleeding oral tissues. This is a common finding in patients with advanced disease, causing physical and/or emotional distress to the patient and caregiver.

Causes

- Candidiasis (thrush): See "Dysphagia and Oropharyngeal Problems" earlier in the section.
- Drugs with antisialogogic (anticholinergic) effects (e.g., tricyclic antidepressants, opioids, antihistamines, major tranquilizers)
- Radiotherapy to the head and neck region
- Dehydration
- Mouth breathing

- Hypercalcemia
- Mucositis

Findings

- Findings are generally self-evident, but the degree of distress to the patient/caregiver may need to be specifically elaborated by open-ended queries and discussion.

Assessment

- Patient and caregiver coping and concerns
- Fluid intake and interest in any type of hydration to relieve symptoms
- Physical examination of oropharynx and skin turgor

Processes of Care

- Tailor therapy to the extent of patient/caregiver concern/distress and specific cause of signs/symptoms if readily ascertained.
- Symptomatic treatment can include use of a room humidifier, ice chips, small sips of water, sugar-free citrus drops, and fruit high in malic acid (apples, pears, nectarines) in patients who can control swallowing and whose airway reflexes are intact.
- Xylitol-based gums can be beneficial in stimulating saliva if the patient is able to chew safely.
- Lemon or lime concentrate in the imitation plastic fruit "squeezers" found in most grocery stores is a low-cost, easy-to-manage aid in symptom management for thirst/dry mouth (stimulates salivation if salivary glands are intact).
- Use of oral swabs with water is helpful, especially to assuage caregivers' concerns or perceptions of a loved one's thirst during the phase of imminent dying. Similarly, application of a petrolatum-based lip balm may prevent lip cracking and be of comfort to those in attendance.
- Pharmaceutical care should be directed at treatment of specific causes (e.g., candidiasis) or attempts to minimize anticholinergic drug use if possible.
- Cholinergic drugs might stimulate saliva from remaining salivary glands in cases where radiotherapy has obliterated the majority of these tissues:
  - Pilocarpine can be used in doses of 5 mg PO, repeated as necessary, or as a 1% to 2% mouthwash.
  - Cevimeline has a longer half-life and can be used in a dosage of 30 mg PO tid.
  - Salivary replacement is possible with commercially available "artificial saliva" preparations.

Goals/Outcomes

- Reduction of physical distress to the patient and psychological distress to those in attendance from associated morbidity

Documentation in the Medical Record

Initial Assessment

- Patient expression of excessively dry mouth
- Physical examination findings: signs of dehydration, lip cracking, mouth breathing, oral candidiasis
- Caregiver coping
- Likely cause of symptoms/signs

Interdisciplinary Progress Notes

- Interventions and results
- Caregiver ability to carry out care and ability to cope

IDT Care Plan

- Specific interventions and follow-up plans

Recommended Reading

Alt-Epping B, Nejad RK, Jung K, et al. Symptoms of the oral cavity and their association with local microbiological and clinical findings—a prospective survey in palliative care. *Support Care Cancer* 2012; 20(3):531–537.

Davies A, Hall S. Salivary gland dysfunction (dry mouth) in patients with advanced cancer. *Int J Palliat Nurs* 2011; 17(10):477–482.

Murphy BA, Gilbert J. Oral cancers: supportive care issues. *Periodontology 2000* 2011; 57(1):118–131.

Plemons JM, Al-Hashimi I, Marek CL, American Dental Association Council on Scientific Affairs. Managing xerostomia and salivary gland hypofunction: executive summary of a report from the American Dental Association Council on Scientific Affairs. *J Am Dental Assoc* 2014; 145(8):867–873.

Sargeant S, Chamley C. Oral health assessment and mouth care for children and young people receiving palliative care. Part one. *Nurs Child Young People* 2013; 25(2):29–34.

Sargeant S, Chamley C. Oral health assessment and mouth care for children and young people receiving palliative care. Part two. *Nurs Child Young People* 2013; 25(3):30–33.

Wolff A, Fox PC, Porter S, Konttinen YT. Established and novel approaches for the management of hyposalivation and xerostomia. *Curr Pharm Design* 2012; 18(34):5515–5521.

Section 4

Appendices

Appendix 1: Palliative Radiation Therapy in End-of-Life Care: Evidence-Based Utilization

Introduction

Palliative radiotherapy is an indispensable tool that can greatly enhance the quality of life in appropriately selected hospice patients with advanced cancer who still have more than a few weeks or months to live. It is primarily used to control pain due to bone metastasis. This form of therapy also can be used to prevent distressing symptoms due to tumor invasion of tissues and organs. In highly selected cases, radiotherapy can allay an "untimely" death from tumor-related hemorrhage, vascular occlusion, or respiratory distress for patients who may not yet have completed their life affairs.

Even in nonhospice environments, it is estimated that about 50% of radiation therapy treatments performed are for palliative reasons like relief of symptoms associated with primary or metastatic cancer. Yet this important form of palliative therapy has not been employed to any great extent in hospice care due to several factors, including cost, inconvenience, and burden to patients, and a lack of understanding on the part of both hospice clinicians and radiation therapists about its utility in this population.

Like all interventions for palliation at the end of life, before embarking upon this form of treatment, the benefits must clearly outweigh risks and burdens. Therefore, hospice clinicians need to understand the potential role for radiation therapy (who, when, what, where, and why). And radiation oncologists need to understand the contextual needs of hospice patients and their caregivers and the system of care under which the final phase of life is being experienced.

Unfortunately, there are few radiation therapy outcome studies that can help direct the care we give to patients with advanced cancer. Much of the practice of radiation oncology is founded upon the personal experiences of therapists, as passed down by their seniors and reinforced through their own practice patterns. Additionally, widely variable approaches are taken to manage similar cases, without well-defined differences in clinical results. These factors prompt the need for critical rethinking in order to provide a basis for rational decision making so that hospice patients may benefit from the appropriate use of palliative radiation therapy.

Ethical Guiding Principles

(adapted and modified from Mackillop, 1996)

• Palliative radiotherapy should be integrated into the comprehensive plan of care.

• The decision to recommend palliative radiotherapy should be based on a thorough knowledge of the patient's circumstances.

• The decision to recommend palliative radiotherapy should be based upon objective information whenever possible, without adding unnecessary suffering or cost to the patient or family.

• The risk–benefit analysis should include consideration of all aspects of the patient's well-being. The short-term risks and benefits of palliative radiotherapy are more important than those that may or may not occur in the future.

• The decision to use palliative radiotherapy should be consistent with the values and preferences of the patient.

• The patient should be involved in the treatment decision to the extent that he or she wishes.

• Time is precious when life is short. Delays and all waiting times should be minimized. Courses of palliative radiotherapy should be no longer than necessary to achieve the therapeutic goal. Science, not individual practice patterns or habits, should guide therapy. Palliative radiotherapy should consume no more resources than necessary.

Indications for Palliative Radiotherapy

• Pain relief
• Bone metastases
• Lung cancer causing chest pain
• Nerve root or plexus compression/invasion
  • Soft tissue infiltration
• Control of bleeding
  • Hemoptysis
  • Vaginal and rectal bleeding
• Control of fungation and ulceration
• Relief of impending or actual obstruction
  • Esophagus
  • Bronchus
  • Rectum
• Shrinkage of tumor mass(es) causing distressing symptoms
  • Brain metastasis
  • Skin lesions
• Prevention of significant functional morbidity and pain
  • Impending bone fractures (long bones, vertebral bodies)
  • Spinal cord compression
  • Superior mediastinal obstruction (e.g., superior vena cava syndrome)

Benefits and Burdens

It takes several days to a few weeks before palliative radiation therapy creates significant therapeutic benefits. Therefore, in order for patients to benefit, they must have a life expectancy of at least 2 to 4 weeks. Patients whose cancer pain is not well controlled by other methods can benefit from palliative radiation therapy. Or, when analgesic therapies create dominant adverse effects, palliative radiation therapy also would be appropriate. These are examples of situations when patients *should be* considered for palliative radiation therapy.

Other times, there are cases where radiation therapy appears to be beneficial but when one views the "opportunity costs" involved, it becomes less desirable. For example, the actual time involved for a patient to receive radiation therapy treatment is short, but the "opportunity cost" shows up in the transport time and associated discomfort the patient experiences. Additionally, the patient experiences waiting time and time away from family, loved ones, and the potentially meaningful activities in which he or she could be participating. All of these factors must be taken into account when weighing the benefits versus the costs of radiation therapy.

Many patients *can* benefit from palliative radiation therapy; simply weigh carefully *all* of the factors when deciding on treatment.

Fractionation

Fractionation schedules (i.e., the number and timing of radiotherapy sessions and the radiation dose[s] per session) for palliative radiation therapy are not yet based upon a firm scientific footing. However, there is much evidence (supported in the following paragraphs) that suggests shorter courses of treatment are just as effective as more protracted schedules. An additional benefit of short courses is they incur less acute toxicity in the patient. With fewer trips to a treatment facility, patients also experience less discomfort and have more time to spend in other endeavors. Additionally, palliative radiation therapy can be costly in comparison to the likelihood of the improved outcomes it may offer.

Bone Pain

Where palliative radiation therapy is indicated, there is much evidence to suggest, under most circumstances, that a short course (one to five doses) is as effective as more protracted treatment schedules (10 to 20 fractions) and incurs less acute toxicity. The most recent clinical trials have strongly suggested that single-fraction therapy is very effective for the treatment of metastatic bone pain.

Non-Small Cell Lung Cancer

The Medical Research Council trials in Great Britain compared a regimen of 17 Gy in two fractions with 30 Gy in two fractions, and a single 10-Gy fraction to the two-fraction treatment in patients with poor performance status (i.e., hospice eligible). The short-course therapy (one or two fractions) proved to be as effective as the longer course approach without incurring any greater toxicity.

Brain Metastases

The data for treating cerebral metastases is similar to that for bone disease. The Radiation Therapy Oncology Group clinical trials and European studies suggest that a three-day course of treatment is as effective as a more protracted regimen.

Fractionation Conclusions

Based upon historical and mounting contemporary evidence, one, two, or a few (at the most) fractions represent the most beneficial approach to palliative radiation therapy, when indicated in patients with limited life expectancy. It would be against the interests of any patient to propose, much less institute, a protracted fractionation schedule that is time-consuming, creates patient discomfort, and is costly in comparison to evidence of the likelihood of improved outcomes compared with a brief intervention.

The approach toward minimal palliative radiotherapy has not yet become the norm in the United States, although it needs to be invoked as a standard of care for hospice patients unless new data emerge to the contrary. Disagreement with such an approach should be challenged on the basis of the scientific evidence, and professionalism in all such discussions should prevail, with a focus on what serves the best interests of the patient.

Acute Toxicity

There are several potential adverse effects associated with radiation therapy. Most develop a week or two after treatment, when tumor cell death is at its peak. These after-effects can be anticipated and should be prevented or treated in order to minimize symptoms.

Fatigue

Frequently, patients voice symptoms of fatigue. The cause of treatment-related fatigue during the actual course of therapy is not well understood. It may be an effect of radiation treatment per se or the exertion required for the patient to attend such therapy.

A brief course of psychostimulants may be a creative and relatively benign means to treat fatigue. As of yet, use of low-dose psychostimulants (e.g., methylphenidate) has not been formally studied for this indication.

Skin Symptoms

The most common finding is localized erythema, which resolves in two to three weeks after completion of therapy. If there is any discomfort associated with it, unbroken skin can be treated with a topical steroid cream (e.g., 1% hydrocortisone). If skin breakdown occurs, this should be treated like any open sore or ulcer (e.g., decubitus care) in order to prevent secondary infection.

Visceral Symptoms

There is a risk of nausea and vomiting during the course of treatment, and these symptoms may persist for a few days following the completion of radiation therapy. Antiemetic therapy should adhere to usual processes of care, starting with first-line approaches (see "Nausea and Vomiting" in Section 3) and progressing to dexamethasone and then ondansetron or granisetron for intractable cases, as necessary.

Diarrhea may occur shortly after exposure of the intestines to radiation therapy. Anticipation of this occurrence by switching to a low-fiber diet (for patients who are eating a full range of foods) may prevent it. If diarrhea does occur, follow established simple processes of care, prescribing loperamide or diphenoxylate as initial therapies.

Dysuria, Urinary Frequency

These symptoms can occur after brief exposure of the bladder to ionizing radiation. Treatment with phenazopyridine and a low dose of an anticholinergic agent (e.g., amitriptyline 10 mg q HS) may provide symptomatic relief.

Conclusion

The sum of the current scientific evidence suggests that palliative radiotherapy continues to be underused in end-of-life care. When it is offered, the frequency of treatment regimens commonly exceeds the likely benefits to be derived, adding greater burden than benefit. An evidence-based understanding and application of its role in symptom management by all health-care providers and caregivers at this crucial time in patients' lives will lead to an improvement in end-of-life care. As with most therapeutic options, appropriate patient selection and informed consent are the foundation of good care. It is now up to hospice professionals and radiation oncologists to act in accordance with the evidence at hand.

Recommended Reading

Ashworth A, Kong W, Chow E, Mackillop WJ. Fractionation of palliative radiation therapy for bone metastases in Ontario: do practice guidelines guide practice. *Int J Radiat Oncol Biol Phys* 2016; 94(1):31–39.

Chow E, Harris K, Fan G, et al. Palliative radiotherapy trials for bone metastases: a systematic review. *J Clin Oncol* 2007; 25(11):1423–1436.

Dennis K, Linden K, Balboni T, Chow E. Rapid access palliative radiation therapy Programs: an efficient model of care. *Future Oncol* 2015; 11(17):2417–2426.

Hartsell WF, Scott CB, Bruner DW, et al. Randomized trial of short- versus long-course radiotherapy for palliation of painful bone metastases. *J Natl Cancer Inst* 2005; 97(11):798–804.

Mackillop WJ. The principles of palliative radiotherapy: a radiation oncologist's perspective. *Can J Oncol* 1996; 6(suppl):5–11.

Mackillop WJ, Kong W. Estimating the need for palliative radiation therapy: a benchmarking approach. *Int J Radiat Oncol Biol Phys* 2016; 94(1):51–59.

Rutter CE, Yu JB, Wilson LD, Park HS. Assessment of national practice for palliative radiation therapy for bone metastases suggests marked underutilization of single-fraction regiments in the United States. *Int J Radiat Biol Phys* 2015; 91(3):548–555.

Tanner C. Palliative radiation therapy for cancer. *J Palliat Med* 2011; 14(5):672–673.

Wai MS, Mike S, Ines H, Malcolm M. Palliation of metastatic bone pain: single fraction versus multifraction radiotherapy: a systematic review of the randomised trials. *Cochrane Database Syst Rev* 2004; (2):CD004721.

Appendix 2 Principles of Pharmacotherapy

General Principles

- Maximize efficacy (therapeutic effect).
- Minimize adverse effects (toxicity).
- Minimize cost (conscious and conscientious resource utilization).
- Know, anticipate, and match pharmacokinetics (what the body does to the drug: absorption, distribution, metabolism, excretion) to the specific circumstances of each patient (age, gender, ethnicity, weight, comorbidities, concurrent drugs).
- Know and anticipate pharmacodynamics (what the drug does to the body: therapeutic and potential adverse or "side" effects) based upon the specific circumstances and characteristics of each patient, including history of drug responsiveness and adverse effects,

Cost–Benefit

- Use generic formulations when this option exists.
- Use more costly formulations only when there is a specific indication.
- Convenience alone (not to be confused with significant issues of compliance) or personal preferences of the prescriber are rarely, if ever, sufficient reasons for medication selection.

Application of General Principles to Opioid Prescribing Practices

- Use the oral or transdermal route unless there are contraindications.
- Contraindications to oral administration: patient is NPO, short bowel syndrome, malabsorption syndrome, dumping syndrome, intractable nausea and vomiting
- Contraindications to transdermal administration: fever, diaphoresis, excessive skin sensitivity, extremes of cachexia or obesity
- Consider the rectal route when oral/transdermal routes are contraindicated, but this is an area where personal issues (patient and caregiver) need to be respected.
- Use continuous/sustained-release formulations for continuous (unremitting) pain.
- Use immediate-release, short-acting formulations for breakthrough pain or for rescue analgesia (more than three or four doses per day should trigger consideration of upward titration of the long-acting formulation).
- Breakthrough pain doses should be from 10% to 20% of the 24-hour dose of total analgesic (e.g., if a patient is taking 60 mg continuous-release morphine by mouth q12hr, the breakthrough pain dose should be about 18 mg [range of 12 to 24 mg] morphine or its equivalent).
- Use alternative or more costly formulations only if there is a specific contraindication to a lower-cost formulation.
- If a patient's pain is well controlled on an analgesic regimen at the time of admission, take a thorough medication history, including past

Appendix Table 2.1 Likelihood of Drug Interactions Occurring with Commonly Used Drugs

Drug Class	Frequent	Occasional	Uncommon
OPIOIDS			
Codeine		*	
Fentanyl			*
Hydromorphone			*
Methadone		*	
Morphine			*
Oxycodone	*		
Tapentadol			*
Tramadol		*	
NEUROLEPTICS			
Haloperidol	*		
Chlorpromazine		*	
ANTIDEPRESSANTS			
Tricyclics	*		
SSRIs	*		
MAO Inhibitors	*		
SNRIs		*	
ANTIEMETICS			
Metoclopramide			*
Ondansetron			*
CORTICOSTEROIDS	*		
BENZODIAZEPINES		*	

reactions/experiences with other opioid analgesics, and change medications only if specific drug-related problems develop.

- Use U.S. Food and Drug Administration (FDA)-approved pharmaceuticals and routes of administration (predictable and proven uptake and absorption) unless there is a clinical need for which there is no approved product available; under these circumstances, compounding is justified. See Appendix Table 2.1 for drug interactions.
- CRITICAL THINKING AND APPLICATION OF SOUND PRINCIPLES OF PRESCRIBING NEED TO BE THE FIRST STEPS OF EVERY MEDICATION ORDER.

Recommended Reading

Chisholm-Burns M, Schwinghammer TL, Wells BG, et al. *Pharmacotherapy: Principles & Practice*, 2nd ed. New York: McGraw-Hill, 2010:3–35.

Fine PG. *Diagnosis and Treatment of Breakthrough Pain*. New York: Oxford University Press, 2008.

Fine PG, Portenoy RK. *Clinical Guide to Opioid Analgesia*, 2nd ed. New York: Vendome Press, 2007.

Appendix 3 Ketamine Protocol

Background

Ketamine is a dissociative anesthetic agent that has analgesic properties in subanesthetic doses. Ketamine is the most potent NMDA-receptor-channel blocker available for clinical use. Ketamine has other actions that may also contribute to its analgesic effect, including interactions with other calcium and sodium channels, cholinergic transmission, noradrenergic and serotoninergic reuptake inhibition and mu, delta, and kappa opioid-like effects. Ketamine also appears to have an antidepressant effect in patients with major depression. Generally, ketamine is used in addition to morphine or an alternative strong opioid when further opioid increments have been ineffective or precluded by unacceptable undesirable effects. When used in this way, ketamine is generally administered PO or SC. It can also be administered IM, IV, SL, intranasally, PR, and spinally (preservative-free formulation).

Indications

- Refractory cancer pain, under the following circumstances:
  - "Maximal" titration of opioid (to include trial of oral methadone) with prior opioid rotation
  - Where side effects of opiates have become a limiting factor in further titration despite opiate rotation
  - Where the oral route for other neuropathic agents is not possible
  - Evidence of opioid-related hyperalgesia
  - Opioid tolerance suspected on basis of rapid escalation of opioid dose without evidence of progressive or new disease
- Ischemic, inflammatory, myofascial pain or severe neuropathic pain where there is unresponsive/limited response to standard therapies
- Painful dressing changes (wounds/burns/ulcers) poorly responsive to other analgesics

Contraindications

- Raised intracranial pressure, epilepsy, severe adverse psychotomimetic effects from ketamine or other past hallucinogenic drug use

Cautions

- Hypertension, cardiac failure, history of cerebrovascular accidents; plasma concentration increased by diazepam

Relative Treatment Exclusions

- Recent psychiatric hospitalization, suicide attempt or ECT in past month
- History of psychosis/schizophrenia
- History of recent seizures
- Uncontrolled raised intracranial pressure due to brain metastases or hydrocephalus

Appendix Table 3.1 Ketamine Continuous Infusion Protocol

	Time (min from start)	Pain score	BP	Pulse	Other	Medications given
Give 0.1 mg/kg IV/SC bolus of ketamine (e.g., 70-kg patient: 7-mg bolus). Reduce opiate infusion by 50%.						
Wait 15 minutes, then monitor.	15					
If good response, consider this dose for basis of infusion; if partial or minimal response, give second bolus at double dose (e.g., 0.2 mg/kg).						
Observe for response over 15 minutes.	30					
If partial response, give third bolus. Maximal dose: up to 0.5 mg/kg, but suggest maximum 20- to 30-mg bolus.	30					
Monitor q15min and observe duration of effective response (usually 15 to 30 minutes but occasionally hours).	45					
Calculate mg/hr rate from duration of response (e.g., if 10 mg lasts 20 minutes, then infusion rate is 30 mg/hr).						
Give additional bolus (at last bolus rate) and then start infusion. Infusion concentration 1 to 5 mg/ml (e.g., If 1 mg/1 ml concentration, run at 30 ml/hr).	50					
May be able to discontinue opiate infusion, but have PCA/bolus opiate available q10-15min						
Reassess in 24 hours:						
Good control: no change						
Titration required: increase infusion rate by 0.05 to 0.1 mg/kg per hour						
Continue to monitor for undesirable psychotomimetic effects, excessive salivation, tachycardia.						

- Severe labile hypertension or poorly controlled cardiac arrhythmia
- COPD with associated hypercarbia

Potential General Side Effects

- Although 40% of patients receiving anesthetic doses via IV/SC route have some side effect, there is a very low incidence of adverse effects reported with subanesthetic doses of ketamine used for pain control. Potential adverse effects include increased oral secretions, hypertension, tachycardia, psychotomimetic phenomena (euphoria, dysphoria, blunted affect, psychomotor retardation, vivid dreams, nightmares, poor concentration, illusions, hallucinations, altered body image), delirium, dizziness, diplopia, blurred vision, nystagmus, altered hearing, and erythema and pain at the injection site.
- Psychotomimetic side effects generally can be controlled by diazepam, midazolam, or haloperidol/chlorpromazine.

Guidelines for Use (SC/IV or Oral)

- Initiation only by approval of Palliative Care Attending
- Use only in care setting with approved policy and procedure or in home setting under physician supervision with informed consent based on benefit-burden discussion with patient and/or proxy.
- Administration/dose escalation by MD or CRNA (under direction of MD) only
- Nurse in charge and assigned to patient has received inservice on ketamine
- Indications for use met and case has been discussed with interventional pain service +/- IDT meeting
- Full collaboration of interventional pain team
- Accurate weight for patient
- Determine patient's prognosis:
  - If short (days to weeks), use continuous infusion (see Appendix Table 3.1).
  - If longer (weeks to months), consider "burst" ketamine (reduces tachyphylaxis/tolerance issues); oral ketamine (see Appendix Tables 3.2 and 3.3).

Appendix Table 3.2 "Burst" Ketamine Protocol SC/IV
Method A (SC)
Initial dose: 100 mg given over 24 hours
Increase after 24 hours to 300 mg/24 hrs if 100 mg is ineffective.
Increase then to 500 mg/24 hrs if 300 mg is not effective.
Stop 3 days after last dose increment.
Method B (IV)
Single 4-hour IV infusion of 0.6 mg/kg

Appendix Table 3.3 Oral Ketamine Protocol

Use direct from vial or dilute to 50 mg/5 ml using flavoring such as Kool-Aid to mask bitterness (i.e., add 10-ml vial of ketamine 100 mg/ml injectable to 90 ml purified water, store in refrigerator up to 1 week).

Initial dose 10 to 25 mg tid or qid and prn

Titrate to optimal effect in dose increments of 10 mg to maximum dose 50 mg qid

Onset of action: 30 minutes; half-life 3 hours ketamine and 12 hours norketamine

Maximum reported dose is 200 mg PO qid.

If hallucinations, mood disturbance, nightmares, or drowsiness occur, give smaller doses more frequently; drowsiness may also improve with reducing opiate by 25% to 50%.

Required Monitoring

- Monitoring required during initial induction period and then q6hr:
  - Vitals: pulse, BP, pulse oximetry
  - Elicit and record pain score.
  - Psychomimetic effects
  - Monitor respiratory secretions.
  - Headaches

Continuous IV/SC Infusion Protocol

Equipment

- Small syringes
- Saline boluses
- Ketamine
- Infusion pump available

Adjuvant Medications Available at Bedside

- Diazepam 5 to 10 mg (seizures unlikely at these doses)
- Chlorpromazine 12.5 to 25 mg q6hr for prevention and treatment of psychotomimetic effects
- Glycopyrrolate 0.2 to 0.4 mg IV/SC for secretions
- Labetalol 2.5 mg q6hr IV for hypertension/tachycardia
- Ketamine is miscible with dexamethasone, diamorphine, haloperidol, metoclopramide, midazolam, and morphine.
- Ketamine can be irritant; dilute in largest volume feasible of 0.9% normal saline.
- Usual dose concentration: 1 to 5 mg/ml

- Inflammation at infusion site can be helped by 1% hydrocortisone cream or by adding dexamethasone 0.5 to 1 mg to the infusion (dilute in 5 to 10 ml normal saline, then add to ketamine).

Recommended Reading

Arroyo-Novoa CM, Figueroa-Ramos MI, Miaskowski C, et al. Efficacy of small doses of ketamine with morphine to decrease procedural pain responses during open wound care. *Clin J Pain* 2011; 27(7):561–566.

Benítez-Rosario MA, Salinas-Martín A, González-Guillermo T, Feria M. A strategy for conversion from subcutaneous to oral ketamine in cancer pain patients: effect of a 1:1 ratio. *J Pain Symptom Manage* 2011; 41(6):1098–1105.

Cohen SP, Liao W, Gupta A, Plunkett A. Ketamine in pain management. *Adv Psychosom Med* 2011; 30:139–161.

Fine PG. Ketamine: from anesthesia to palliative care. *AAHPM Bull* 2003; 3(3):1–6.

Jackson K, Ashby M, Martin P, et al. "Burst" ketamine for refractory cancer pain: an open-label audit of 39 patients. *J Pain Symptom Manage* 2001; 22:834–842.

McCaffrey N, Hardy J, Fazekas B, et al. Potential economic impact on hospitalisations of the Palliative Care Clinical Studies Collaborative (PaCCSC) ketamine randomised controlled trial. *Aust Health Rev* 2015 (epub ahead of print).

Slatkin NE, Rhiner M. Ketamine in the treatment of refractory cancer pain: case report, rationale and methodology. *Support Oncol* 2003; 1(4):287–293.

Appendix 4 Clinical/Functional Assessment and Staging

Appendix Table 4.1 Palliative Performance Scale (PPS)

%	Ambulation	Activity and Evidence of Disease	Self-Care	Intake	Level of Consciousness
100	Full	Normal activity, no evidence of disease	Full	Normal	Full
90	Full	Normal activity, some evidence of disease	Full	Normal	Full
80	Full	Normal activity with effort, some evidence of disease	Full	Normal or reduced	Full
70	Reduced	Unable to do normal work, some evidence of disease	Full	Normal or reduced	Full
60	Reduced	Unable to do hobby or housework, significant disease	Occasional assistance necessary	Normal or reduced	Full or confusion
50	Mainly sit/lie	Unable to do any work, extensive disease	Considerable assistance required	Normal or reduced	Full or confusion
40	Mainly in bed	As above	Mainly assistance	Normal or reduced	Full, drowsy, or confusion
30	Totally bed bound	As above	Total care	Reduced	Full, drowsy, or confusion
20	As above	As above	Total care	Minimal sips	Full, drowsy, or confusion
10	As above	As above	Total care	Mouth care only	Drowsy or coma
0	Death	–	–	–	–

Adapted with permission from Anderson G, Downing M, Hill J, Casorso L, Lerch N, Palliative Performance Scale (PPS): A New Tool. Journal of Palliative Care 1996;12(1):5–11. Copyright: Institut universitaire de gériatrie de Montréal.

New York Heart Classification: A Clinical Guide

Stage I heart disease: No symptoms of heart disease (Palliative Performance Score [PPS] 100) (see Appendix Table 4.1)

Stage II heart disease: Symptoms of heart disease at MORE than normal activity (PPS 80)

Stage III heart disease: Symptoms of heart disease at LESS than normal activity (PPS 60)

Stage IV heart disease: Symptoms of heart disease at REST or at MINIMAL activity (PPS ≤ 50)

Functional Assessment Staging

The Functional Assessment Staging Tool (FAST) is a useful means of codifying far-advanced dementing illness, and it has some prognostic value as a component to hospice eligibility determination under current provisions of the Medicare Hospice Benefit. It was published as Reisburg B. Functional assessment staging (FAST). *Psychopharmacol Bull* 1988; 24:653–659 and can be located at: http:www.acsu.buffalo.edu/~drstall/fast.html.

Eastern Cooperative Oncology Group (ECOG) Performance Status

These scales and criteria are used by doctors and researchers to assess how a patient's disease is progressing, to assess how the disease affects the daily living abilities of the patient, and to determine appropriate treatment and prognosis. They are included here for health-care professionals to access. (See Appendix Table 4.2.)

End-Stage Liver Disease

The Model for End-Stage Liver Disease (MELD) is a scoring system for assessing the severity of chronic liver disease. It was initially developed at the Mayo Clinic to predict death within three months of surgery in patients who had undergone a transjugular intrahepatic portosystemic shunt (TIPS) procedure, and was subsequently found to be useful in determining prognosis and prioritizing for receipt of a liver transplant. This score is now used by the United Network for Organ Sharing (UNOS) and Eurotransplant for prioritizing allocation of liver transplants instead of the older Child-Pugh score.

Calculation

MELD uses the patient's values for serum bilirubin, serum creatinine, and the International Normalized Ratio for prothrombin time to predict survival. It is calculated according to the following formula:

$$MELD = 3.78\left[Ln \text{ serum bilirubin } (mg/dL)\right] + 11.2\left[Ln \text{ INR}\right]$$
$$+ 9.57\left[Ln \text{ serum creatinine } (mg/dL)\right] + 6.43$$

$$(Ln = natural \ logarithm)$$

UNOS has made the following modifications to the score:

• If the patient has been dialyzed twice within the last seven days, then the value for serum creatinine used should be 4.0.

Appendix Table 4.2 ECOG Performance Status

Grade	ECOG
0	Fully active, able to carry on all pre-disease performance without restriction
1	Restricted in physically strenuous activity but ambulatory and able to carry out work of a light or sedentary nature, e.g., light house work, office work
2	Ambulatory and capable of all self-care but unable to carry out any work activities; up and about more than 50% of waking hours
3	Capable of only limited self-care, confined to bed or chair more than 50% of waking hours
4	Completely disabled. Cannot carry on any self-care; totally confined to bed or chair
5	Dead

Reprinted with permission from Oken MM, Creech RH, Tormey DC, et al. Toxicity and Response Criteria of the Eastern Cooperative Oncology Group. Am J Clin Oncol 1982;5: 649–656.

The ECOG Performance Status is in the public domain therefore available for public use. To duplicate the scale, please cite the reference above and credit the Eastern Cooperative Oncology Group, Robert Comis M.D., Group Chair.

- Any value less than 1 is given a value of 1 (i.e., if bilirubin is 0.8, a value of 1.0 is used) to prevent the occurrence of scores below 0 (the natural logarithm of 1 is 0, and any value below 1 would yield a negative result).

Patients with a diagnosis of liver cancer will be assigned a MELD score based on how advanced the cancer is.

Interpretation

In interpreting the MELD score in (hospitalized) patients, the three-month mortality is as follows:

- 40 or more: 71.3% mortality
- 30–39: 52.6% mortality
- 20–29: 19.6% mortality
- 10–19: 6.0% mortality
- <9: 1.9% mortality

Appendix 5 Anticoagulation

Several conditions encountered in advanced illness care require consider-ations about use of anticoagulants in order to prevent morbidity or prema-ture mortality. The two main categories are oncologic conditions and patients with atrial fibrillation. (See Appendix Tables 5.1 and 5.2.)

- **Cancer:** There is an established relationship between cancer (CA) patients and venous thromboembolism (VTE).
  - CA patients maintain a hypercoagulable state.
  - Thrombotic events are the second leading cause of death in CA patients.
  - Anticoagulants are indicated for all high-risk CA patients (if appropriate within the goals of care).
    - Untreated deep venous thromobosis (DVT) increases risk of pulmo-nary embolism (PE) by 50%.
    - Recommended length of anticoagulation therapy and specific therapy are not fully defined by evidence.
    - Side-by-side superiority drug investigations are not inclusive of CA patients.
- Advanced CA patients maintain pro-thrombotic tendencies and indefinite treatment is generally recommended.
- There exists a greater risk of death from acute PE relative to fatal bleeds from anticoagulation.
- Anticoagulated CA patients have an elevated incidence of major bleeds (about 13% higher than untreated patients) regardless of specific type of anticoagulation therapies.
- **Atrial Fibrillation:** Atrial fibrillation (AF) is a prevalent condition in older patients, averaging about 5% of this population, and twice that in patients with symptomatic coronary artery disease, valvular heart disease, and/ or heart failure. Since patients with AF are at high risk of embolic stroke, most patients with chronic AF will be treated to prevent this devastating complication (see Appendix Fig. 5.1).
- **Goal of Anticoagulation:** Minimize risk of DVT, PE, and stroke while managing the risk of a major bleed.

Appendix Table 5.1 Injectable Heparin Therapies

Drug	Category	Indication	VTE Prevention Dose	Monitoring Parameters	Renal Impairment Indications*	Emergent Reversal Agents	Costs per day
Lovenox (Enoxaparin)	Low-molecular-weight heparin	DVT and PE prophylaxis and treatment	40 mg SQ daily	Periodic; platelets, occult blood, anti-Xa levels, serum creatinine	Reduce to 30 mg daily if Clcr < 30 ml/min	Hold drug, dose-dependent protamine	$72.83
Fragmin (Dalteparin)	Low-molecular-weight heparin	DVT and PE prophylaxis and treatment	5,000 units SQ daily	Periodic; CBC/PLT, occult blood	$T_{1/2}$ increases with chronic renal failure by 40%. Dose modification with Clcr ≤ 20 ml/min	Hold drug, dose-dependent protamine	$182.92
Arixtra (Fondaparinux)	Factor Xa inhibitor	Treatment (no indication for prophylaxis with medical patients)	>50 kg = 2.5 mg SQ daily	Periodic; CBC/PLT, occult blood	Dose modification with Clcr < 50 ml/min	Hold drug, dose-dependent protamine	$104.45
Unfractionated Heparin	Anticoagulant	DVT and PE prophylaxis and treatment	5,000 units SQ twice daily	Platelet counts should be routinely monitored (e.g., every 2 or 3 days on days 4–14 of heparin therapy) and hemoglobin, hematocrit, signs of bleeding; fecal occult blood test; aPTT	Adjust to therapeutic aPTT	Hold drug, dose-dependent protamine	$4.00

AF: atrial fibrillation; VTE: venous thromboembolism; DVT: deep venous thrombosis; PE: pulmonary embolism; Clcr: creatinine clearance; CBC: complete blood count; PLT: platelets; LFT: liver function tests; HCT: haematocrit; PT: prothrombin time; PTT: partial thromboplastin time; aPTT: activated partial thromboplastin time; INR: international normalized ratio; TT: thrombin time; ECT: ecarin clotting time.

Appendix Table 5.2 Oral Anticoagulants

Drug	Category	Indication	Dose	Monitoring Parameters	Renal Impairment Indications*	Emergent Reversal Agents	Cost
Coumadin (Warfarin, Jantoven)	Vitamin K antagonist	DVT and PE prophylaxis and treatment AF stroke reduction **Significant drug–drug interactions and related contraindications**	Titrated to effect	*PT/INR, HCT Goal: 1.5 to 2.5 (frequency varies on INR stability) Potentially useful (limited): CBC/PLT, aPTT	Increased risk of bleeding complications with renal failure	Withhold drug, high-dose phytonadione, consider clotting factor supplement: PCC4, PCC4 + PCC3 + rFVIIa, aPCC, PCC3, rFVIIa, FFP	Cost: ~.58/tablet >$600/annually PT/INR testing
Pradaxa (Dabigatran)	Anticoagulant, thrombin inhibitor	DVT and PE prophylaxis and treatment AF stroke reduction **Significant drug–drug interactions and related contraindications**	150 mg PO twice daily	aPTT values >2.5× control may indicate over-anticoagulation Potentially useful (limited): Scr, CBC/PLT, INR/PT, aPTT, TT, ECT, dilute TT	Dose modification with Clcr 15 to 30 ml/min 75 mg/BID (Pradaxa should not be used with more than one bleeding risk factor, to include Clcr <30 ml/min)	Withhold drug, give activated charcoal if dosed <2 hours prior or HD for >2 hours ago. Consider clotting factor: aPCC, PCC4, PCC4 + PCC3 + rFVIIa	$10.00 (tablets)
Xarelto (Rivaroxaban)	Factor Xa inhibitor	DVT and PE prophylaxis and treatment AF stroke reduction Contraindicated with severe hepatic impairment **Significant drug–drug interactions and related contraindications**	20 mg PO daily *with food in patients with Clcr >50 ml/min*	Periodic CBC/diff & PLT, Scr, and LFT Potentially useful (limited): PT/INR, chromogenic antifactor Xa assay	AF: CrCl 15 to 50 mL/min 15 mg once daily with the HS with meal Contraindicated with Clcr <15 mL/min *VTE Prophylaxis:* Contraindicated: Clcr <30 ml/min	Withhold drug, give activated charcoal if last dose given <2 hours prior and repeat 6 hours after last dose. Consider clotting factor supplement: PCC4, aPCC, PCC4 + PCC3 + rFVIIa, or PCC3	$10.50/day

Eliquis (Apixaban)	Factor Xa inhibitor	DVT and PE prophylaxis and treatment AF stroke reduction Contraindicated with severe hepatic impairment	5 mg PO twice daily	Potentially useful (limited): Scr, CBC/PLT, PT/INR, chromogenic antifactor Xa assay	AF: 2.5 mg twice daily if patient has two or more of risk factors (age ≥80, weight ≤60kg, SC ≥1.5mg/dL) 2.5 mg twice daily if co-administered with strong inhibitor of CYP3A4 and P-glycoprotein. Contraindicated with two PLUS risks AND taking a strong dual CYP3A4 and P-gp inhibitor. No data to support use with Clcr <15 ml/min *VTE Prophylaxis:* 2.5 mg twice daily	Withhold drug, give activated charcoal if last dose given <2 hours prior and repeat 6 hrs after last dose. Consider clotting factor supplement: PCC4, aPCC, PCC4 + PCC3 + rFVIIa, or PCC3	$10.00/day
Edoxaban (Savaysa)	Factor Xa inhibitor	DVT and PE treatment ONLY AF stroke reduction Contraindicated with severe hepatic impairment	60 mg once daily in patients with Crcl >50 to ≤95 ml/min	Limited usefulness: PT and aPTT	30 mg once daily in patients with Clcr 15 to 50 mL/min Contraindicated in patients with Clcr >95 ml/min	No specific antidote Edoxaban is not dialyzable	$11.00/day

** All regimens have literature supporting accumulation with impaired renal function and advanced age; monitoring for signs and symptoms of bleeding is essential.

AF: atrial fibrillation; VTE: venous thromboembolism; DVT: deep venous thrombosis; PE: pulmonary embolism; Clcr: creatinine clearance; CBC: complete blood count; PLT: platelets; LFT: liver function tests; HCT: haematocrit; PT: prothrombin time; PTT: partial thromboplastin time; aPTT: activated partial thromboplastin time; INR: international normalized ratio; TT: thrombin time; ECT: ecarin clotting time.

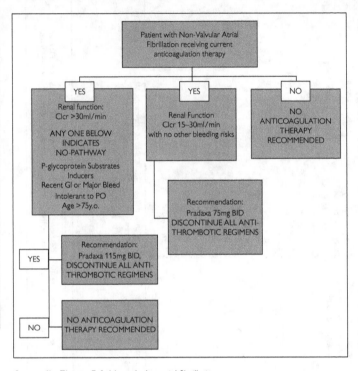

Appendix Figure 5.1 Nonvalvular atrial fibrillation

Treatment Recommendations

High-Risk Malignancy and Risk of VTE

- Mucin-producing adenocarcinomas (see Appendix Figure 5.2)
- Pancreatic CA
- Gastrointestinal tract CA
- Lung CA
- Ovarian CA
- Or as determined by the medical director or oncologist
- And consistent with the patient's plan of care

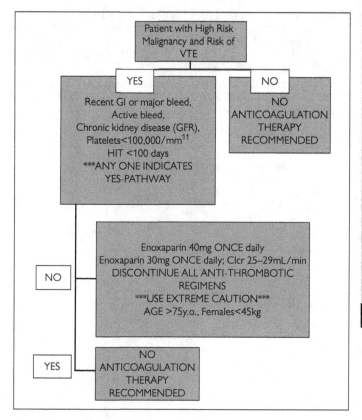

Appendix Figure 5.2 High-risk malignancy and risk of VTE

Recommended Reading

Le Maître A, Ding K, Shepherd FA, et al. Anticoagulation and bleeding: a pooled analysis of lung cancer trials of the NCIC Clinical Trials Group. *J Thorac Oncol* 2009; 4(5):586–594.

Lexi-Comp Online. *Lexi-Drugs Online*. Hudson, OH: Lexi-Comp, Inc., 2010. http://online.lexi.com/ (accessed January 10, 2016).

Lyman GH, Khorana AA, Kuderer NM, et al. Venous thromboembolism prophylaxis and treatment in patients with cancer: American Society of Clinical Oncology clinical practice guideline update. *J Clin Oncol* 2013; 31(17):2189–2204.

Mahan C, Spyropoulos A. ASHP therapeutic position statement on the role of pharmacotherapy in preventing venous thromboembolism in hospitalized patients. *Am J Health System Pharm* 2012; 69:2174–2190.

Noble S, Shelley MD, Coles B, et al. Management of venous thromboembolism in patients with advanced cancer. *Lancet Oncol* 2008; 9(6):577–584.

Nutescu EA, Dager WE, Kalus JS, et al. Management of bleeding and reversal strategies for oral anticoagulants: clinical practice considerations. *Am J Health Systems Pharm* 2013; 70:1914–1929.

Perez A, Eraso LH, Merli GJ. Implications of new anticoagulants in primary practice. *Int J Clin Pract* 2013; 67(2):139–156.

http://www.uptodate.com/contents/search?search=anticoagulation+guidelines (accessed January 10, 2016) [multiple articles and guidelines on anticoagulation].

Index

Tables, Figures and boxes are indicated by an italic *t*, *f* or *b* following the page number, respectively.